When You're **HOT,** You're **HOT**

Also by Jan King

Hormones from Hell
It's a Mom Thing
It's a Girl Thing

When You're **HOT,** You're **HOT**

How I Laughed My Way Through Menopause

Jan King

Andrews McMeel Publishing

Kansas City

To my wonderful girlfriends who courageously fought
and won their battles with cancer:

Carlynn Donosky, Jane West, Kathy Buckley, Elizabeth Jackson,
Marilyn Taylor, and Margaret Larmon

and

In memory of my beloved friend who lost hers,

Linda Wexler

02 03 04 05 RDH 10 9 8 7 6 5 4 3 2

Library of Congress Cataloging-in-Publication Data
King, Jan.
    When you're hot you're hot : how I laughed my way through menopause / Jan King.
        p. cm.
    ISBN 0-7407-2222-0
        1. Menopause—Humor. 2. Middle aged women—Health and hygiene—Humor. I.
    Title.

RG186 .K54 2002
612.6'65—dc21

2001056180

Book design by Holly Camerlinck
Cover photograph by Charles William Bush
Hair by Carolyn Carroll
Makeup by Jus' Judy
Nails by Marla Burgess

Contents

Acknowledgments

To my husband, Mark, thank you always for your love and your continued support in sickness and in health.

To my editor, Kelly Gilbert, whose insight and understanding of this field, especially for a young gal, constantly amaze me. Even though I am old enough to be your older sister, I won't hold that against you.

To my friend Jon Anderson, thank you so much for your guidance and friendship. I think you are truly one of the brightest men in this business.

To my mom and dad, to Karen and Bob, Paul and Ginny, Michael and Whitney, and Philip, you'll never know how much your love and support mean to me. You were all instrumental in helping me make a complete recovery.

To my doctors, Sharon Winer, Philomena McAndrew, Gary Tearston, Herbert Stein, Joseph Lebovic, and Mitchell Karlan, you made all the difference in my successful treatment and recovery. Thank you for giving me back my life, which is, now, better than ever.

Introduction

Well, girls, a lot of estrogen has passed under the bridges of Menopause County since I wrote *Hormones from Hell.* Since then, I have had a big change of life—in more ways than one. I am happy to announce that I have successfully gone through menopause. Yep, that's right. I'm officially out of the egg business.

You can count on me to give you the real scoop about the metamorphosis your middle-aged body will be going through. And trust me, you won't be getting a sugarcoated placebo. I'll deliver the real thing.

Actually, it's quite a chic time to be going through menopause, for you're in the company of such luminaries as Cybill Shepherd, Bette Midler, Lauren Hutton, and Suzanne Somers. I don't think Cher has gone through menopause, though. In fact, I don't think she'll ever go through it. The only thing she'll go through is another surgery. She looks like she's still thirty. Maybe a little waxy, but definitely sexy. But you've got to hand it to her. After all that singing about turning back time, she actually did it.

When You're Hot You're Hot will answer some hard-hitting, James Carville–type questions like: Is there life after menopause? Can we learn to cope with sagging skin, irritable bladder syndrome, and sleepless nights? Can we make some sort of attractive centerpiece out of all those unused tampons sitting in our bathroom closets?

Well, if you are getting seriously depressed about all of this female stuff—don't. Just throw back an Ensure shooter with a Pepto-Bismol chaser while you read my book. In no time, you'll be laughing and feeling much better.

When you're finished, I promise you'll feel good enough to come busting out of your menopausal closet. And speaking of closets, you can get a lot of straightening done in yours . . . while you're up all night . . . between bathroom runs.

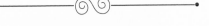

But Seriously . . .

A Woman's Worst Nightmare

It's sometimes hard for me, as a humorist, to tell just the truth. The truth is, I had a tough time, as you'll learn throughout this book, dealing with the onset of my menopause and developing and fighting breast cancer. But I survived, more or less intact, with a healthy body, a good firm grip on reality, and, thank God, my sense of humor.

So this book is a bit of a departure from my others. Don't worry, I haven't stopped telling jokes, but through these "But Seriously . . ." sidebars, I am also going to pass on a lot of the knowledge I gained from surviving this difficult period. Hopefully, you'll learn some valuable things from my experience, and that knowledge will make a difference in your lives.

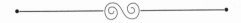

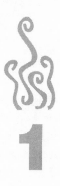

POWER SURGES:

Sweatin' with the Oldies

Call me nuts. I've heard it before. The fact is that I am probably the only woman in the world who enjoyed going through menopause. Yep. You heard me right. Why? Because menopause is the only time in life when a woman can get away with all kinds of rude behavior—including murder. Not long ago, I read about a case where a woman killed her husband, then pleaded not guilty because of temporary insanity brought on by menopause. And she won the case. Crazy? Yeah, like a fox.

Wow! Just think of the possibilities this opens up to us, considering that menopause lasts roughly 1.4 centuries. Okay. I exaggerated. 1.2 centuries. But here's the thing. Before menopause, I was always the calm decision maker, the peace broker, the voice of reason—you know, traditional woman stuff. But once it got started—and I embraced the possibilities—I found that I had a huge window of time to complain, carry on, and act like a total bitch. I could make everybody around me as miserable as I was feeling. And here's the best part. Nobody blamed me. They just shook their heads and said, "Go easy on her. The poor woman is going through the change, you know."

Crimes of Hormones

Perp	The Crime	The Time
Lorena Bobbitt	Cut off husband's penis and threw it in a field	$25 fine for littering
Betty Broderick	Stalked and shot ex-husband and new wife	$100 fine for hunting out of season
Patrizia Reggiani	Ordered Mob hit on cheating husband, Maurizio Gucci	Six months of anger-management classes
Christine English	Ramming boyfriend into utility pole with her car	Eight-hour course at driving school
Dorothea Puente	Poisoned six boarders with arsenic	One month of community service on poison-control hot line

So for the first time in my life, I could be as obnoxious as I wanted to be *and* garner sympathy in the process. I'd say that was cause for celebration. Premarin's on the house!

I found that if I thought of menopause like a pregnancy, it became okay for me to indulge myself without feeling guilty. I slept till noon. I cried an ocean. And while we're on the subject of saline, I busted open that twenty-six-gallon bag of salty chips I bought at Costco. Why not? I was already retaining more water than the Hoover Dam. What's a few more pints? Believe me, I know how hard it is to accept going through the change. In the beginning, I had a devil of a time facing reality. Compared to me, Farrah Fawcett on *Letterman* had a better grip on reality.

Diary of a Really Mad Housewife

Menopause was spitting in my face like an Egyptian cobra, but I was floating on DeNile. How blind could I be? My body was giving me more signs than Sidney Omar's tarot cards, but I wasn't reading any of them.

Night 1: November 3, 1992—a day that will live in infirmary. I wake up at 3 A.M. with a body so hot, you could cook a Lean Cuisine on it. My nightie is drenched with sweat and plastered flat across my chest (or across my flat chest—either is technically correct). The bedroom is freezing, thanks to the electric company's Antarctic Energy Savings Plan my husband signed up for.

But it doesn't make any difference. I am generating a hormonal heat wave so intense, steam is rising off my body. The two fronts collide, creating a thunderstorm directly above my bed. Yet, I am sweltering. I push off the covers and fall back to sleep.

An hour later, I wake up encrusted in a layer of my own frozen sweat. I look like a modern-day mastodon preserved in permafrost. It's official: I am on the brink of extinction.

Night 2: A repeat of the one before. This time, I blame it on my flannel pj's. In my semiconscious state, I experience a Larry Flynt–type revelation, except I do not come face-to-face with Jesus in a private jet 37,000 feet above the earth. Instead, I come face-to-face with Larry Flynt himself. He prophesies that I will incinerate the pages of *Hustler.*

Nights 3 through 7: I am out of excuses. What could it be? Let's see. I am forty-eight years old, skipping periods, and suffering through mood swings that occur roughly every six seconds. I go from Donna Reed to a cop-slugging Zsa Zsa before you can say "plea bargain."

I ask myself over and over, "What does this mean?" Du-uh. (What it means is that it's high time for a reality check.) Instead, I convince myself that I have a terminal disease. Right. It's called terminal denial.

Day 8: I must see a doctor. I consult my ob-gyn, and her

diagnosis rocks my world. You got it—menopause. My youth is going down faster than a White House intern. Bummer. I immediately go into mourning for my lost youth. I have visions of myself sporting lavender-tinted hair and playing bingo at the local VFW. Worse yet, I will be labeled with foul names like "Grandma" and "senior citizen."

Day 9: I sit quietly trying to collect my thoughts. But I am interrupted by the whine of my triceps sagging and the skin on my neck crinkling up. I look into the mirror and notice I have developed jowls and a bunch of stray chin whiskers. I not only feel as ornery as a pit bull, but I am beginning to resemble one.

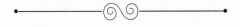

But Seriously ...

Perimenopause

This is really roughly what happened to me, except the most urgent reason I sought help from my gynecologist was that my periods were out of control. They were interfering with my daily life. I would skip a period one month, and then the next I'd be bleeding so heavily that I couldn't leave my house for two days.

A pelvic sonogram and uterine biopsy determined that a thickened uterine lining was causing the heavy bleeding. This is one of the most common occurrences during perimenopause. I began a regimen of low-dosage birth control pills to correct the problem.

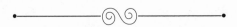

Day 10: I need more knowledge about this milestone event all of us baby boomers are collectively experiencing. Translation: Misery loves company.

I hit the information highway, and logged on to www. overthehill.com. Along with Al Gore's résumé, this is the information I found:

World Stats

Year 2000: 50 million women in the world over fifty
years of age
Year 2020: The number will increase to 60 million.
Year 2025: 30 percent of the world's female population
will be menopausal.

Although I feel somewhat comforted by these statistics, I know on the other hand that this is really bad news for Julio Iglesias.

The Pits

Here's the list of the top ten symptoms of menopause as I experienced it:

1. Hot flashes
2. Heart palpitations
3. Headaches
4. Memory loss
5. Water retention
6. Decreased bladder control
7. Vaginal dryness
8. Loss of sex drive
9. Erratic mood swings
10. Depression—Gee, I wonder why

Did I list memory loss? I forget.

Doctors prescribe hormone replacement therapy (HRT) to alleviate the hot flashes and mood swings during menopause. But it also has a lot of side effects like even more bloating and irritability. Oh, great. Just what we need. A "cure" that keeps on giving. Now we'll be reeling around like a loose cannon for another ten years. I am convinced that HRT is a medical code for "Having a Rough Time."

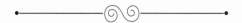

But Seriously …

Reducing the Risks

The uncertainty of when my periods were going to occur forced me to cancel a lot of the travel necessary to promote my books. I was not in control, and I was not happy. My doctor felt that low-dosage birth control pills would be a good way to control my heavy periods. The other option was to have a D & C, which would only take care of the problem temporarily. During perimenopause, a woman is still producing hormones, but at a reduced rate. The birth control pills turn off ovulation, thus giving you a more steady state of hormone production. My gynecologist felt that this was safe for me because I was a healthy, nonsmoking woman.

She did tell me that one of the possible side effects was blood clots. A small percentage of the population carries a genetic predisposition to blood clots. So Dr. Winer had me take a blood test that would predict whether my body had the tendency to form clots.

This test was done back in 1995, and it's not a test your gynecologist does routinely. However, if you are in a high-risk category for blood clots, there are about six tests available today that your doctor can choose from. Mine came back negative, so we went ahead with the low-dosage oral contraceptives.

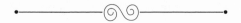

BLOAT

So forget the top ten symptoms of menopause. BLOAT is a Jan acronym that identifies the syndrome and the state of your body for the next decade:

B for "bugged." You're menopausal as hell and aren't going to take it anymore. Everyone around you has an attitude problem. However, your hostility is aimed mainly at two groups:

1. Perky, cute women under thirty with thin ankles and flat abs.
2. All perky, cute women under thirty.

L for "losing it." During menopause you will lose total control over . . .

1. your body temperature
2. your emotions
3. your bladder

O for "oversensitivity." Bursting into tears over issues of global importance like . . .

1. unsightly panty lines
2. split ends
3. those darn cellulite bumps

A for "argumentative." Impossible to look at your husband anymore without picking a fight. Accompanied by an irresistible urge to strangle him with your underwire bra. (Note: Retain an attorney and cop a PMS plea.)

T for "tired." From having to get out of bed four times a night to relieve a bladder that at some unknown point in time has shrunk down to the size of a walnut.

Well, girls, there it was. I thought I could handle it. I took solace in the fact that I wasn't alone. Millions of my sisters were crying, sweating, and cursing along with me.

These days, menopause is on everyone's mind. The whole world has become menopausally enlightened. The population has been prepared for our forgetfulness, our mood swings, and our tirades. If you don't believe me, just tune in to PMSNBC, the world's angriest network. Watch nasty women broadcast daily crisis reports and continuously bitch and moan about our condition. So, I relaxed. I enjoyed myself. I went out and beat up a Cabbage Patch Kid.

Menopause: The Good News and the Bad News

The good news: Your family treats you to a series of seminars.
The bad news: In anger management.

The good news: You get time to spend the entire day on the phone.
The bad news: With the suicide hot line.

The good news: Since you can't get pregnant anymore, you are having the best sex of your life.
The bad news: You can't remember having it.

The good news: You don't have to wear those bulky sanitary pads.
The bad news: You have to wear those bulky Depends.

The good news: There is no longer a need for your husband to get a vasectomy.
The bad news: He wants one anyway.

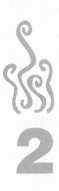

PMS:

Next Mood Swing Six Seconds

Oh, great. Just what I don't need. More misinformation about menopause. Now, the experts are saying that as menopause approaches, many women will develop PMS *for the first time*. Helloooo. Where have these experts been living all their lives—in their freezers?

Get a life. I started having PMS back in high school before they even named it. Come on. We all did. And it could become pretty severe at times. Where do you think they came up with the plot for the movie *Carrie*?

Public Enemy Number One

We're all familiar with teenage "attitude." In my day, I gave as good as I got. No big mystery here. It's not a matter of poor parental discipline. It's just PMS rearing its ugly head. And like older women, many teenage girls suffer with depression and frequent crying spells. They have mood swings, anxiety, and periodic bouts of rage. Those poor kids. Is it any wonder that Alanis Morissette and Fiona Apple are their idols? Talk about your angry chicks. These young women have forged a career out of it. God help them when they mellow out after menopause. Their careers are history.

But when you really think about it, why shouldn't they be pissed and moody? Do the math. Out of thirty days, they spend seven premenstrually bloated. Then it's followed by seven more days of having a period accompanied by headache and cramps. But wait. There's still another seven days of postmenstrual depression. My God. They're lucky to get five good minutes a month! And get this—during menopause it gets worse! Wait until you experience your first hot flash. You'll be sitting there, cool as a cucumber one minute, then you'll turn beet red and start sweating profusely the next. Not only that—now your periods will become more irregular than Dick Cheney's cardiogram. You'll never know when they're going to happen, or what to expect when they do.

There is an upside, though. Nowadays, it's acceptable to blame everything from a bad personality to a homicide on PMS. Women have roughly thirty years to cry, throw tantrums, and even assault somebody without penalty. That's some hat trick, huh?

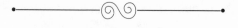

But Seriously . . .

A Natural Tranquilizer

Mood swings are the natural fallout of hormonal changes during the life span of any woman. They're inevitable. However, I have discovered a miracle mood elevator, and it's not a pill. It's exercise. I work out six times a week doing aerobics and kick-boxing classes. No matter how angry or depressed I am when I enter the gym, after thirty minutes of exercising, these oppressive feelings lift. I always leave the gym feeling happy and centered. I was able to handle menopause and breast cancer with no Valium, Xanax, or any other tranquilizer. Natural endorphins are my quick fix. I believe that my exercising regimen was a crucial part of my successful recovery.

Psychology of Hormones

The following psychological conditions are allegedly the result of hormone imbalances:

Social Anxiety Disorders

Psychiatrists believe that fluctuating hormones may be the culprits in many anxiety-related disorders. Many of them arise during menopause. Some women report experiencing panic attacks that seem to come out of nowhere, accompanied by heart palpitations, sweating, a fear of losing control, and an overwhelming desire to flee the scene. Gee. Sounds familiar. This used to happen to me on most of my dates. I just didn't know what it was back then.

As a result of panic attacks, some women become afraid to leave their homes. The name for this condition is agoraphobia. Literally translated from the Latin, it means "fear of the marketplace." Gosh, I have that too. Come to think of it, most Americans do. Especially when they hear that Alan Greenspan is raising interest rates.

But not to worry. The drug companies have manufactured a new generation of drugs that successfully treat anxiety disorders. One of the most popular is called Paxil. Currently, millions of people are taking it. I don't understand why it's so popular, though. The side effects are worse than the panic attacks. You can develop diarrhea, nausea, and cotton mouth. If you ask me, I think you're better off staying at home, alone, with a couple of martinis.

Obsessive-Compulsive Disorder (OCD)

For people afflicted with OCD, simple behaviors like handwashing and straightening furniture can become the focus of their lives. They may repeat one action for hours. OCD can transform you from a dream housewife into your husband's worst nightmare. I'm just glad I don't have it. How do I know? My psychiatrist told me. I called him twenty times one day to make sure.

OCD is a psychological condition that is becoming rampant in our society. Many menopausal women fall victim to OCD.

They find themselves with a compulsion to keep repeating simple behaviors over and over again. And if they don't go through the rituals, they suffer great anxiety.

Maybe our society is to blame for creating and perpetuating these social disorders. Back in my parents' day, it seemed like nobody had these problems. They were too busy trying to make a living. They didn't have time to indulge themselves in fruitless behaviors. But now, it's different. My husband and I are more affluent. We have more leisure time. We're drinking Starbucks coffee all day, so we're up all night. Then we're so tired we get depressed, and we have to start taking Prozac. Then we get on our cell phones, because we can't stop talking about it. I guess we're living in a world that practically ensures we're all going to become neurotics.

It makes me wonder whether all of us pre- and post-menopausal women are really nuts—or is society just making us appear that way? Well, I, for one, think I'm pretty darn normal. Just last week at my alien abduction support group, one of the gals told me how together I was.

Clinical Depression

Contrary to medical opinion, I think it's perfectly normal for women to cry a lot. And there's no need to keep taking happy pills and medicating ourselves into a stupor, either. I'm okay, you're okay.* The real problem lies in our culture. We live in a society that expects everyone to act perky and enthusiastic all the time. Give me a break. Where is it written that we have to act like some freakin' contestant on *The Price Is Right* twenty-four hours a day? If you ask me, I say all this happiness is not normal.

When I was a kid, it seemed like nobody's mom was happy. But it was okay with them. They never felt like they needed medication, either. Being grouchy and moody was accepted as a normal state of life. Honest. All of my female relatives were pretty depressed most of their lives. There was a rumor that my grandmother actually smiled once in 1955, but it's still unconfirmed.

* It's the psychiatrists who are nuts.

It's reassuring to know we're not going crazy. It's our hormones doing this to us. We don't need Prozac. The truth is that depression is a normal state. Happiness is just a chemical imbalance.

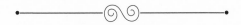

But Seriously ...

Getting a Grip

I was diagnosed with lobular breast cancer during menopause, and my gut reaction was overwhelming fear. When that wore off, I spent two hours crying about it. Then I got depressed and angry, because I felt so victimized. Totally normal. Most women go through all these stages just coping with menopause.

I started meditating once a day for twenty minutes. My meditation plus my exercise regimen helped me gain control over all of these emotions. It works, trust me. I used to dismiss meditation as some "New Age" foolishness. But no more. It helped me handle and even eliminate much of the stress in my life. Practiced daily, I find that it provides an inner peace that no drug could ever give me.

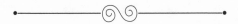

As a menopausal woman, I can understand why we're not running around jumping for joy. When I went through the change of life, I had a lot to be upset about. What kind of things? Can you give me a few days? No? Well, let me give you the short list of things that get my panties in an uproar:

Cellulite

Hot flashes

Massengill commercials

Kathie Lee Gifford

Cody and Cassidy

Any correspondence from the AARP
Early bird specials
Carmen Electra
Anything or anybody on MTV

PMS Rage

This is a hormonally driven condition in which a woman experiences uncontrollable anger. It can be so severe that she is capable of committing a homicide during this fugue state. Nowadays we read about women who have killed their husbands during PMS rages. However, most of them get acquitted because their lawyers can enter a plea of temporary insanity from PMS.

As if this wasn't bad enough for the husbands, get this—they haven't found a medication to prevent the rages yet. So watch your backs, guys. If I were a man married to a menopausal woman, I'd confiscate any of her possessions that could be used as a lethal weapon. This includes her underwire bras, her garter belt, her acrylic nails, and her frozen pot roast.

I know one thing. If I ever get arrested for a PMS crime, I'll never be able to pull off a good defense. Even if they told me I had the right to remain silent, I just wouldn't be able to quit talking. I'd probably blab myself right into the electric chair.

Mad About You

So I've gotten angry and yelled a lot, so what? It's not a syndrome, it's part of regular life. PMS or no PMS, I've done my share of screaming around my house. In fact, I sounded like a Yoko Ono album for almost two decades.

I don't see anything wrong in blowing your stack every once in a while. An occasional fight can be very therapeutic. Oh, come on. Admit it. Doesn't it do your soul good to go ballistic every now and then? The problem is that doctors keep telling us that it's not normal. They consider it pathological.

Really? The behavior of guys like John McEnroe, Bobby Knight, and Puff Daddy is considered normal. Even admirable.

Dennis Miller has a hit show on HBO based on his infamous "rants." And the more he rants, the more the public loves him. Men like these are called "macho," "heroes," and "powerful" by our misguided society. However, if a woman acts like this, they say it's because our hormones are making us crazy. We are branded as "nut jobs," "bitches," and "loose cannons."

But this just isn't so. During menopause, something cataclysmic occurred in my brain. What happened was that for the first time in my life, I began to say what I really thought, not what I thought people wanted to hear. Maybe it's psychological. Or maybe it's because the brain cells responsible for censoring speech died off from hormone intoxication. But it's most likely because I was producing a lot more testosterone, so I actually grew some balls.

Anger management? Why can't my husband understand that? I'm not an unreasonable woman. I've always believed marriage was a give-and-take proposition. I give the orders and he takes them. What's wrong with that? But nowadays, if I act even a little aggressively, I'm told I need to take anger-management classes. Forget it. I tried counseling, and you know what? It ruined my fighting skills.

Case in point: If my husband got drunk at a party and flirted with some tart, I'd be really steamed. Before anger management, I would have retaliated with this bombastic speech:

"You moron! I'm sick and tired of you acting like a total jerk when you get drunk. You spent half the night at the bar, flirting with that ugly old bag. Who the hell do you think you are? Well, you're no Mel Gibson, that's for sure. Face the facts, buster. You're fat, bald, and impotent. If you don't start acting your age and showing me some respect, I'm going to kick your sorry butt to the curb."

But after attending anger-management classes, this is the tirade I'm supposed to deliver:

"You mentally challenged person! I have issues with your alcohol intolerance. It makes you act like you're psychologically impaired. You spent all night conversing with that aesthetically impaired, chronologically and morally challenged female. You are not Jesse Jackson. You're a horizontally and follicularly challenged man who is also sexually impaired. I'm recommending therapy in hopes that your emotional age will catch up with your chronological age. If you do not seek therapy, I will have no other recourse but to retain legal counsel and terminate this marriage. Have a nice day."

That went well, didn't it? Oh, pul-leeze. This politically correct ka-ka will get you nowhere. It's like pitting Pewee Herman against Mike Tyson. Society has to learn that it shouldn't mess with a fifty-something menopausal maven.

I have entered the stage in my life when my hormones are giving me power surges that rival an electric company's.* I no longer have to march to the beat of someone else's drum. I am marching to the irregular beats of my own menopausal heart.†

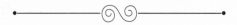

But Seriously . . .

Fear of Feelings

Men seem really insensitive to our feelings a lot of times, especially during menopause. But that's because they really don't have a clue as to how much havoc our hormones wreak on our bodies. Sometimes a man's gut reaction is anger, but it really masks fear. Men get scared when they see their normally stoic wives losing some control.

When I was first diagnosed with breast cancer, my husband and I reacted by having a series of little squabbles. It was because we both felt that the security and control we had worked so hard for was being blown apart. But we kept talking and working through it, and when I was facing bilateral mastectomy surgery and really needed his support, he was there for me 100 percent.

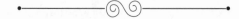

* Except Con Ed in California.
† To the anthem "I Am Woman, Hear Me Roar."

. Quiz .

Hormonal Horrors

1. The role model for menopausal women that has best endured the test of time is . . .
   a. Gloria Steinem
   b. Cybill Shepherd
   c. Hillary Clinton
   d. Lizzie Borden

2. One of the better therapies for treating menopausal aggression is . . .
   a. Prozac
   b. Paxil
   c. Elavil
   d. obedience training

3. During menopause, the best source for your medications is . . .
   a. the pharmacy
   b. your gynecologist
   c. natural herbs
   d. Darryl Strawberry

4. Panic attacks happen most frequently when . . .
   a. you're driving
   b. you're in an unfamiliar place
   c. you're in a crowd
   d. you open your Nordstrom's bill

5. The herb most commonly taken to reduce aggression in menopausal women is . . .
   a. Saint John's-wort
   b. kava-kava
   c. ginko biloba
   d. marijuana

6. Jewish people have always used this term of endearment when referring to their menopausal women:
    a. bubbeleh
    b. balabusta
    c. maven
    d. meshuggener

7. The most common affliction that can put a menopausal woman behind bars is . . .
    a. PMS
    b. OCD
    c. ADD
    d. DUI

Quiz Results

The answers to all of the above are d, as in "delusional."
    1–3 correct: Behavior modification therapy recommended.
    4–7 correct: Continuous Prozac IV drip—stat!

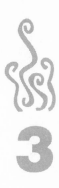

3

MENOPAUSAL MAINTENANCE:

Used Parts

For best results, you'll need to get in the mood to read this chapter. So, follow my instructions. Sit down in a comfortable chair. Great. Now, prop your legs up. No, farther. Straight up in the air . . . that's right. Are they in geographically different zip codes? Good. Now you're ready to begin. Oh, yeah. Did I mention, you should be naked from the waist down?

Aw, don't take it so hard. This is going to be pretty much your state of being for the next decade. When going through menopause, I did some serious bonding with my gynecologist. My existence was dedicated to the care and maintenance of body parts that showed more wear than a Kmart sheet. And speaking of sheets, that's what I was wearing for much of my menopausal stretch. I underwent more tests than a lab rat at SmithKline & French.

Six Feet from Hell

The medical tests I received during menopause ranged from the relatively simple to the incredibly humiliating. And they all had this one thing in common: *They were performed with an instrument that is a six-foot flexible tube with a light and/or camera attached to the end.*

This instrument is one scary piece of equipment. It looks just like a plumber's snake. It also performs similar functions—like reaming, probing, and repairing small leaks. No wonder our reproductive systems are commonly referred to as "female plumbing"!

I'm going to cut through all the bull, and give you the real story about the medical tests I experienced going through menopause. You will not get a euphemized, sanitized version like you'd expect to hear from your health-care provider—who used to be called your doctor in the old days, in case you forgot. No siree, Bob. These stories are not for the squeamish. You'll probably get weak in the knees. So fasten your stirrups. You're in for a bumpy ride.

The Gynecology Exam: A Deeper Look

The examination. I was asked to take "everything off" and put on one of those horrid examination gowns. These gowns are not exactly designed by the House of Dior, either. They are especially designed to provide minimum coverage with maximum exposure by . . .

   . . . barely covering my ovaries

   . . . making my tushie hang out through the six-inch gap in the back

The gyno exam is always given on a steel examination table in a room that has never gotten above thirty-two degrees. So besides suffering from menopause, I added frostbite to my list of complaints.*

I quickly discovered that during the first visit, it was a smart move to present my gynecologist with a head shot of myself. That's because it would be the first and last time she'd ever see my face. From then on, all our conversations took place with her head under the sheet, talking directly into my cervix.

The procedure. The gynecologist performed a manual exam-

---

* Technically, frost*butt.*

ination of my cervix and ovaries. She also did a "Pap smear" at this time. This is a simple test in which the cervical cells are scraped and fixed on a slide for biopsy.

I was not alone in the room. A nurse or physician's assistant was always present during the examination. Nowadays, the doctors have to do this to protect themselves against lawsuits.* You can always tell the doctors who have been sued in the past. Besides the nurse, they also have a courtroom stenographer present in the examination room.

But wait, there's more. A group of new interns also showed up on their rounds. These guys looked so young, many looked like they hadn't gone through puberty yet. We're talking peach fuzz and pimples here. I also noticed that they had replaced their clip-on ties with stethoscopes to make themselves look more credible. They spent a good fifteen minutes furiously taking notes and drawing intricate diagrams of my uterus with their box of forty-eight Crayolas.

At this point, I might as well have invited the entire secretarial pool, cleaning crew, and anyone else out there to come in and have a look, too. Why deny anybody? Like childbirth, menopause is an occasion in which the concept of modesty is totally eradicated from your world. Our "private parts" have officially become *public domain*.

The results. My doctor called me in about a week with the results. I was not at home, so my husband took the message. He told me that my doctor called, but he couldn't remember what she said. Just that he thought it had something to do with "Pabst beer."

Endometrial Biopsy

The examination. Because I was experiencing such heavy bleeding with my irregular periods, my doctor needed to look at the cells in my uterus and see if there were any growths causing it. She took a piece of tissue from my endometrium (lining of the uterus) and had it examined under the microscope. Any removal

---

* They always wear gloves to avoid leaving fingerprints.

and examination of tissue is called a biopsy. A cytologist (cell specialist) in a lab then examined the slide for abnormalities in my uterine cells. The biopsy also revealed a lot about my hormone levels, which were now plunging faster than Roger Ebert on a bungee.

The procedure. This test is similar to a Pap smear except that the tissue is endometrial rather than from the cervix. This means that the doctor must go higher up in the uterus to get it. How does she do that? How else? That good ol' six-foot flexible tube. The tube is narrow enough to be pushed up through the cervix into the uterus. Sounds bad. But don't panic yet. It takes a while to get there. I was lying there thinking, "Uh-oh. If she goes up any higher, she's going to extract a wisdom tooth."

The tube is small enough to accomplish the procedure without the use of an anesthetic. I was told that it would produce some "mild discomfort"—like menstrual cramps. What she didn't tell me was the menstrual cramps she was referring to were those of an elephant. So whenever you hear the words "mild discomfort"— watch out! It's medical double-talk for "Call an anesthesiologist."

The results. The tissue samples were "fixed" on slides, and then sent off to a lab, where they were instantly misplaced. The lab called me with a lame excuse, trying to blame their screw-up on my doctor. No matter who got blamed, the result was the same: I had to go back and have the whole procedure repeated a week later.

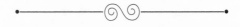

But Seriously . . .

A Little Pain / a Lot of Gain

An endometrial biopsy can provide some potentially life-saving information. It can detect abnormalities in the uterine cells that a Pap smear would miss because that test only collects cells from the cervix. An endometrial biopsy collects from the uterine lining. It gives the doctor a lot of information about your hormone levels, and how far you are into menopause.

My doctor advised me that irregular bleeding or even light spotting should never be ignored or considered "normal" for menopause. Even though I kid about it, this procedure was really fairly painless and can be performed in your doctor's office. It's truly not a big price to pay for the potentially life-saving information it gives your doctor.

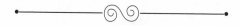

The Transvaginal Pelvic Sonogram

The examination. This is another procedure that falls into the general category "naked from the waist down." This one is performed by a radiologist in his or her office. I had it done because my gynecologist wanted to see how thick the lining of my uterus had become, and whether that could be causing my heavy bleeding.

The sonogram utilizes sound waves to give an extremely accurate picture of internal organs. The radiologist looks for cysts, tumors, and/or calcifications in the uterus and ovaries. He or she also accurately measures the thickness of the uterine lining, which in my case, was suspected as the source of my heavy bleeding.

The procedure. The radiologist, Dr. Lebovic, used a long, wandlike instrument with a rolling ball-like part that was passed over the exterior of my pelvic area. The sensation was actually quite pleasant. I told myself, "Go ahead—relax! Enjoy that fantasy about Gustav, the hunky masseuse at the gym." Hmmmm. It actually felt good. But I shouldn't have gotten so comfortable. That innocuous little wand did a magic trick, and presto change-o! It elongated into a periscope, probing deep into my interior parts, searching for the enemy.

This was not, repeat, not the time to be fantasizing about Gustav and his magic fingers. No way. This was the time for a full-blown epic like *Saving Private Ryan.** This new sensation was more like a German tank blasting its way through the Uterine Alps.

* More like *Saving Ryan's Privates.*

The result. The doctor was able to view the interior of my uterus in real time on a monitor in the examination room and immediately print out my results. He also immediately printed out my bill—to the sonic tune of $300.

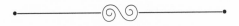

But Seriously . . .

Nip It in the Bud

When you're going through menopause, I think it's a good idea to pay closer attention to your uterus and ovaries. Because of fluctuating hormones, it's a time when the lining of the uterus often thickens, causing heavy bleeding. We also have to be watchful for other changes, including possible endometrial or cervical cancers. A pelvic sonogram is an excellent diagnostic tool to keep a watchful eye on things.

A transvaginal pelvic sonogram is able to detect even the tiniest cysts, growths, or changes in the uterine lining or ovaries. If he or she does find any changes, it will be in plenty of time to do something about it, before it becomes a real problem. I have this test done yearly, because I take a drug as part of my breast cancer treatment that increases the chance of getting uterine cancer. Most doctors will recommend a pelvic sonogram if you have irregular bleeding or to detect ovarian tumors.

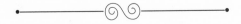

The Sigmoidoscopy

The examination. After I turned fifty, my internist recommended I start having a sigmoidoscopy every two to three years. This is an examination of the sigmoid colon, the last part of the large intestine. The "sigmoid" is done by a medical specialist called a proctologist. Unfortunately, these doctors are the subject of more butt jokes than Jennifer Lopez.

The procedure. The sigmoidoscopy is performed with an instrument called a sigmoidoscope that . . . Take a wild guess. Another six-foot flexible tube with a light and/or camera attached to the end? That's right, Quincy. The doctor asked me to lie on my side, and inserted the sigmoidoscope into an area anatomically known as the bootie. Then he booted it up and headed on up my ten-inch colonic highway. He looked at the inside of my colon on a monitor, searching for polyps, tumors, or inflammation.

To get a really good view, he had to pump air into my colon while he was probing. But let me tell you something. The colon has a big problem with being treated like a helium balloon. It reacts by cramping and trying to force the air back out. This is when I got all spastic on the table. It was so painful, I think the procedure should be called pump and jump.

The result. By the end of the procedure, I was left with a belly full of air and some pretty big cramps. But the law of physics states that what goes in must come out. So when he retracted the sigmoidoscope, I prayed that I wouldn't start sailing around the room like an inflatable doll that had just had its cork pulled.

The Colonoscopy

The examination. When the *entire* length of the colon is examined, it is called a colonoscopy. This procedure was brought to national attention when Katie Couric had it done, live, on network TV. Way to go, Katie! She heroically and unselfishly did it to raise public awareness.* My proctologist felt I needed this test when I turned fifty-five years of age just as a routine procedure. Also, my chances of colon cancer are slightly higher now that I have had breast cancer. Man, oh, man. Do the perks never end?

The procedure. The worst part is the "prep" for the test the day before the procedure. I was forced to drink approximately one hundred gallons of fizzy, lemony stuff, called "Go-Litely." It should

* And her Nielsen ratings.

be called "Go-Carefully" because just getting an ounce of this stuff down made me gag like a cat with a giant hair ball. Basically, it's the world's most powerful laxative. How powerful is it? Think "scud missile enema," and you're in the ballpark.

Warning. I spent the next twenty-four hours in my bathroom. And once I was there, I also needed to wear a seat belt while sitting on the john.

The result. I hoped that if my colon shots were good enough, I might be approached by HBO for a special. I could forget network. Katie and her ratings-grabbing colon got there first.

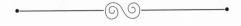

But Seriously...

Another Tool for Early Detection

The colonoscopy is the best diagnostic tool we have to discover any kind of hidden problem along the entire length of the large intestine. And the beauty of this test for me was that I was totally asleep during the entire process. I couldn't believe it when the nurse woke me and said it was over!

Proctologists recommend that anybody over fifty have this done once every five years. I personally know two women my age who had cancers detected during this exam. The great news was that after their tumors were removed, neither needed chemotherapy because the colonoscopy revealed the presence of the tumors in such early stages that only their surgical removal was necessary.

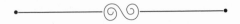

The Mammogram

The examination. I think we are all familiar with the mammogram, an X-ray of the breast to determine whether any tumor is present. My only question is: Who thought up that name? It sounds as though you should put stamps on your breasts and mail them someplace.

The procedure. I always had my mammograms done in a clinic or doctor's office that offered the latest model of low-dosage X-ray machine—the Chernobyl 2000. The technician positioned my breast on a metal tray, like a lamb for slaughter. Then she pulled down a lucite plate with so much force that my breast got flatter than an IHop flapjack.

I was told not to breathe when she repeated it for the side view. Oh sure. Who has any breath left when your breasts are being steamrolled? When the mammogram was finished, I practically had to roll my breast up like a fruit wrap to get it back into my bra.

The result. The nurse had me sit in the waiting room until the radiologist read my results. Realistically, I knew this meant anytime between 9 A.M. and 5 P.M.—or sometime before the next solar eclipse.

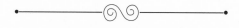

But Seriously . . .

Mammograms Aren't Foolproof

Mammograms can detect up to 85 percent of breast cancers. The good news is that they can find many tumors when they are still so small that you can't even feel them during a manual examination. But the bad news is that mammograms still miss 15 percent of breast cancers. This happened to me. My mammogram didn't show my tumor. This was because lobular cancer, which is what I had, often doesn't form micro-calcifications as do the more common ductal cancers, and these microcalcifications are very visible on a mammogram.

If I hadn't been as conscientious as I was about doing monthly self-exams, my tumor could have gone undetected for months. By then it would have spread significantly, and probably become life-threatening.

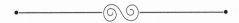

Okay, I think we're done here. My goal was to make you a lot more knowledgeable about the medical aspect of menopause. I know what you're thinking, though. You're thinking, "What makes her such an expert? Should I be taking medical advice from a woman who writes humor books for a living?"

The answer is—of course you should! I may not be a doctor, but I was married to one for twenty years. And that gave me the license* to misdiagnose all my friends on a daily basis for over two decades. God, I was good!

Anyway, when it comes to menopause, who should know better? Me, a respected author, or some guy who's the target of a million butt jokes?

---

* From the College of Barbers and Surgeons.

·Quiz·

Compliments of the Marquis de Sade

1. The most important quality your gynecologist should have is . . .
   - a. a good bedside manner
   - b. board certification
   - c. ten or more years of surgical experience
   - d. a glove size of 6 or less

2. Do not use a gynecologist who recommends having a Pap smear . . .
   - a. every five years
   - b. once every six months
   - c. before the age of eighteen
   - d. with a general anesthetic

3. The mammogram technician was incompetent if you leave with . . .
   - a. blurred X-rays
   - b. painful breasts
   - c. incomplete results
   - d. radiation burns

4. The most common cause of pelvic pain is . . .
   - a. menstrual cramps
   - b. ovarian cyst
   - c. pelvic inflammatory disease
   - d. tight Levis

5. What appliance is not kept in a gynecologist's office?
   - a. coffee maker
   - b. autoclave
   - c. centrifuge
   - d. bun warmer

6. You have taken the correct amount of Go-Litely when . . .
   a. your bowel is evacuated
   b. you feel bloated
   c. you're gagging uncontrollably
   d. you look like beef jerky

7. In the armed services a proctologist is called . . .
   a. a major
   b. a colonel
   c. a general
   d. a rear admiral

Quiz Results

The answers to all of the above are d, as in "Don't touch me!"

   4–7 correct: You're in a good position.

   1–3 correct: You need a leg up.

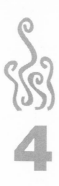

MENOPAUSAL LINGO:

Get a Good Buzz On

Menopause is like an adventure into an exotic country. Which country? Oh, let's say Bosnia. And who better to conduct this menopausal trek than moi. Been there, done that. I've had many years of dealing with the problems in that foreign land. Okay, I may not be any Condoleezza Rice, but I'm no Slobodan Milosevic, either.

I felt the best way to prepare myself for this journey was to become familiar with the lingo—i.e., the native tongue of my doctors. These guys are experts at giving complicated names to simple conditions. For example, when I went to my doctor with a simple bellyache, he refused to call it just that. Instead, he said I might have colitis, ileitis, or pancreatitis. So now, besides experiencing pain, I was experiencing confusion, too. But that's their art. The truth is that they're all better spin doctors than medical doctors.

But take heart. I am going to lift you out of this menopausal miasma and make you more enlightened than the Dalai Lama. After mastering the scientific terms, you can throw them into your everyday conversation. You'll have your audience spellbound with your command of medicalese. Besides, they'd have to be nuts to walk away from a menopausal woman who's in the middle of a massive mood swing.

You'll be casually dropping esoteric names like "phyto-chemical," "luteinizing hormone," and "endometrium" in every conversation. At last you'll be able to understand the technical terms for feeling like *&$%!!

So, get ready for your vocabulary lesson. I'm also going to give you a break, and make Menopause 101 really easy to understand. I will give you a simplified definition and a synonym or derivation of each word. You're not going to get some phony spin-doctor explanation, either. As you know, most of our human anatomy has Latin names. But not to worry. I studied Latin and biology in college, so trust me, I know what I'm talking about. For example, the word "cesarean" literally translated means "salad with anchovies."

Okay. Are you ready? Let's get buzzed.

Jan's Mixed-Up Menopausal Dictionary

Chasteberry

Medical definition: A natural herb used to decrease mood swings and irritability.

A.k.a.: Medieval marijuana.

The scoop: Centuries before PMS was a recognized syndrome, this herb was smoked by the entire population. As a result, everybody sat around eating junk food, and no one showed up for the Seventh and Eighth Religious Wars.

D & C (Dilation and Curettage)

Medical definition: A surgical procedure in which the cervix is dilated and the uterus is scraped with a curette, to obtain cells for biopsy.

A.k.a.: "Dig and cut."

The scoop: The surgeon dices and slices your uterus with the same dexterity a chef would use to fillet a mignon. The question is whether there's going to be enough of your uterus left for it to still qualify as a bona fide organ or only as an hors d'oeuvre.

Don Quai

Medical definition: A Chinese herb used to alleviate the hot flashes and irritability accompanying menopause.

Chinese translation: Donkey.

The scoop: An appropriate name, because those menopausal hormones have you acting like a jackass.

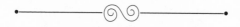

But Seriously ...

Medicinal Herbs

There are millions of women who feel that natural herbs are just as effective as and safer than prescription drugs. This may or may not be true. However, there is one thing that we need to be aware of. Herbs may be natural, but it doesn't mean that they are totally safe for everyone or can be taken in any quantity.

There are many products sold under the heading of "herbs" that are not FDA approved and have not been tested for purity before they are put on the market. So just be aware of this and use caution when taking any supplement. Check with your doctor first. Many have side effects by themselves or in combination with other drugs that the public isn't aware of. For example, even vitamin E, for all the good it does, can cause bleeding problems in some people if taken in large quantities.

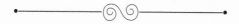

Endometrium

Medical definition: The lining of the uterus. After menopause, the endometrium no longer is sloughed off and menstruation ceases.

Latin derivation: Endo = "end." *Metrium* = "cotton." Literal translation: "Good-bye, Tampax."

The scoop: Your period stops. So, big deal. Who's going to miss it? If you ask me, any woman who still wants a baby after menopause should have her head examined, not her uterus.

Estrogen

Medical definition: The master female hormone. When it decreases, during menopause, symptoms develop such as headache, breast tenderness, nausea, bloating, and weight gain.

Latin derivation: Estrus = "end of." *Genus* = "life." Literal translation: "Touch me and I'll kill you."

The scoop: Be afraid. Be very afraid. Approach with caution. It's easier to negotiate with a woman carrying a load of ammo than one who's light on estrogen.

Fibroids

Medical definition: Benign tumors of the uterine wall, causing uterine enlargement. They can grow so large that a woman may mistakenly believe she's pregnant.

Derivation: From the Old English word "*fibre*," meaning "a bun in the oven."

The scoop: The first symptom is having to exchange your 501 Levis for 1002's.

Flush

Medical definition: The rush of blood, usually in the face and the neck, accompanying a hot flash.

Latin derivation: From the phrase "*tempis flushus*," meaning "my life is going down the aqueduct."

The scoop: Menopausal women are no longer going down the drain. We're back in control. Thanks to Prozac and the spin doctors, nowadays, we're experiencing *power surges.*

Follicle-Stimulating Hormone (FSH)

Medical definition: This hormone stimulates an egg to mature each month in the ovary. Then the egg ruptures through the ovarian wall and begins its journey through the fallopian tube, heading toward the uterus. This process is called ovulation.

A.k.a: FSH stands for "*f*eeling *s*hitty and *h*orrible."

The scoop: The side effects are—what else? Bloating and nausea, the cornerstones of a woman's life. From now on, the only good years you'll have will be the ones on your car.

Free Radicals

Medical definition: Highly reactive molecules implicated in aging and disease.

A.k.a.: Wait a minute! Weren't these a bunch of rabble-rousing hippies in the seventies?

The scoop: The bad news is that not only do we have to deal with them now, but we used to date them.

Hormone Replacement Therapy (HRT)

Medical definition: Hormones given during menopause to boost dwindling amounts of estrogen and progesterone.

A.k.a.: HRT stands for "*h*aving a *r*otten *t*ime."

The scoop: Do we really need to take chemicals that make us more bloated, more depressed, and more prone to blood clots? The therapy is so risky, you'd get better odds with a lottery ticket.

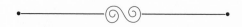

But Seriously . . .

It's Still Your Decision

Although a link between HRT and breast cancer has been highly publicized, at this point in time, most of the doctors I know still feel that HRT does not cause breast cancer. Dr. Winer says that forty years of experience and several major studies suggest strongly that there is no statistical evidence yet showing that HRT causes breast cancer. However, if you already have undetected breast cancer and begin HRT, it can promote the tumor's growth. Doctors and researchers estimate that most breast cancers take eight to fifteen years to diagnose from the first cell changes.

My personal advice is to always keep in mind that this is their opinion, and not the word of God. As more medical evidence comes into existence, often these opinions change. I recently read a study published in the newspaper that said if you have fibrocystic breast disease and are on HRT for more than five years, your chances of getting lobular breast cancer (the type I had) are eight times greater than normal. However, many of these studies published today are controversial, and the results may be skewed. So you should trust your doctors, but also follow your own intuition about your body.

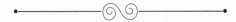

Hot Flashes

Medical definition: The effects of decreased estrogen on the hypothalamus, or sweating and flushed skin.

A.k.a.: "*Highly flammable.*"

The scoop: Hot flash? That's the understatement of the year. You could spontaneously combust at any minute.

Hypothalamus

Medical definition: The area of the brain responsible for regulating body temperature.

Latin derivation: Hypo = "under." *Thalamus* = "water." Literal translation: "I'm drowning in my own sweat."

The scoop: The average body temperature of a menopausal woman is approximately 380 degrees Fahrenheit. Give me a break. I don't even bake a cake in an oven that hot.

Incontinence

Medical definition: During menopause, the muscles surrounding the urethra weaken, resulting in the inability to control urine flow.

A.k.a.: The Oooops Moment.

The scoop: There comes a time in life when we can't even laugh, cough, or sneeze without soggy results. So if we can't laugh, we might as well cry. Is it any wonder we're moody and depressed 99 percent of the time?

Menopause

Medical definition: The state in which the body's production of hormones has decreased to the point where menstruation and pregnancy are impossible.

Latin derivation: Meno = "man." *Pause* = "terminate." Literal translation: "You are the weakest link—good-bye!"

The scoop: When a woman can no longer become pregnant, men become biologically useless. Our sexual interest in them comes to a screeching halt. Technically, men have two remaining functions:

1. Lawn maintenance
2. Auto repair

Osteoporosis

Medical definition: Menopausal bones thin out and weaken because of the reduction of normal calcium absorption.

A.k.a.: "I've fallen and I can't get up."

The scoop: The first sign of osteoporosis is when your panty hose doubles as a tube top.

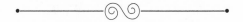

But Seriously ...

Lost: Bone Mass

Bone loss can become a problem after menopause. But the good news is that nowadays, we are really vigilant about osteoporosis and can do something about it. Most doctors recommend a bone-density test for women and men over fifty. It's painless, easy, and can be performed in your doctor's office.

A bone-density test will very accurately tell whether you have suffered any bone loss and how much. If you are losing bone density, your doctor may prescribe extra calcium and a regimen of weight-bearing exercise. The newer drugs used in the prevention and treatment of osteoporosis help to increase calcium absorption. One of the new drugs given to post-menopausal women is called raloxifine (brand name Evista). It has the added bonus of protecting against breast cancer, too.

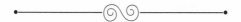

Perimenopause

Medical definition: The hormonally influenced period that precedes actual menopause. It's like having a long siege of PMS.

A.k.a.: PMS stands for "*p*issed-off, *m*oody, and *s*wollen."

The scoop: So far there hasn't been a drug invented that can make us feel good. Wait a minute. This just in . . . Experts say marijuana is being sold to help women suffering from PMS. Now, there's a drug deal you don't want to go bad!

Progesterone

Medical definition: The hormone that gradually turns off estrogen receptors during menopause, causing PMS, memory loss, hot flashes, and food cravings.

Latin derivation: From *Progesterosaurus*, a giant prehistoric lizard that was known to sweat profusely, cry intermittently, eat everything in sight, and then promptly forget about it.

The scoop: I don't know about you, but I kind of enjoy having PMS. It's the only time when I can really be myself.

Saint-John's-Wort

Medical definition: A herb used in the treatment of depression.

Derivation: It was discovered in Russia and has been manufactured there for centuries.

The scoop: Judging by the Russian sense of humor, the herb obviously doesn't work. The only thing more depressed than the people is the economy.

Sepia

Medical definition: A substance obtained from the ink of cuttlefish, purported to alleviate vaginal dryness and increase the sex drive.

A.k.a.: Sold under the trade name "Viagra of the Sea."

The scoop: The squid was unavailable as a spokesperson, so they got Bob Dole instead.

Testosterone

Medical definition: The male hormone that promotes the growth of facial hair, lowers the voice, and increases aggressiveness and sexual drive.

Latin derivation: From *Testosterus*. Literal translation: "Big head, small brain."

The scoop: The good news: With menopause your sex drive increases. The bad news: Your husband's decreases now that you look more like Marilyn Manson than Marilyn Monroe.

Vaginal Dryness

Medical definition: A condition in which the vaginal walls thin and dry out as a result of decreased estrogen production.

Derivation: From the American Indian phrase *"vaginchockta,"* meaning "woman with buffalo bottom."

The scoop: During menopause, there are more women drying out than at an A.A. convention.

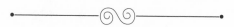

But Seriously...

"Know Yourself"

It is always in our best interest to educate ourselves better, medically. Knowledge is power. The more you know about the way your body works, the more attuned you'll become in detecting and understanding how to treat its problems.

Learn as much as you can about menopause. It will be invaluable in helping you to make better decisions about your treatment. You will better understand what your doctor is talking about, and this in itself helps reduce the dread associated with going through it. Then you can proceed more rationally. The same holds true if you are diagnosed with a disease or other medical condition. You could ultimately save your own life.

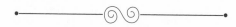

So there you have it. My unabridged, unapproved dictionary of medical terms. Study them and you, too, can be an expert. Once I suffered a hot flash at a dinner party and some well-intentioned old biddy said, "What's the matter with you? You're sweating like that freshly roasted pig on the platter." I calmly turned to the ignoramus and ripped off this riposte:

"My dear lady. I am experiencing a power surge, formerly known as a hot flash. It is caused by the decrease of estrogen and progesterone in the corpus luteum. At the same time, my FSH values are dangerously increasing. But don't get your panties in an uproar. I'm taking a prescribed regimen of HRT and phytochemicals administered through a transdermal patch. It will help alleviate the symptoms caused by this temporary fluctuating hormonal condition."

By the time I finished delivering this epiphany, the old bat had fallen asleep with her face in her soup. She could just as easily have hanged herself from the chandelier.

Either way, I was a winner.

So, surge away, gals!

· Quiz ·

Buzz-Word Bingo

1. Caroline Warmus murdered seven men during a menopausal rampage. Women will always think of her as . . .
   a. psychotic
   b. menopausally homicidal
   c. schizophrenic
   d. a role model

2. How can you tell if you have a prolapsed bladder?
   a. Your doctor diagnoses it.
   b. You get frequent infections.
   c. You're in constant pain.
   d. You're reading this in the bathroom.

3. Which medical procedure has been permanently banned on menopausal women?
   a. cesarean section
   b. oophorectomy
   c. sterilization
   d. cloning

4. When Queen Elizabeth went through menopause, the press described it as . . .
   a. a private matter
   b. being indisposed
   c. an annus horribilis
   d. a royal flush

5. The herbs chasteberry, Saint-John's-wort, and blessed thistle can all be purchased at . . .
   a. a health-food store
   b. the pharmacy
   c. a holistic center
   d. a Catholic church

6. A certain group of menopausal women who are treated like queens by men and have gifts lavished on them are called . . .
   a. tribal elders
   b. sages
   c. beloved wives
   d. mistresses

7. The ancient Roman statesman who was considered the father of modern birth control was . . .
   a. Julius Caesar
   b. Marcus Aurelius
   c. Lucius Andromicus
   d. Coitus Interruptus

Quiz Results
The answers to all of the above are d, as in "direct current."
  1–3 correct: Short circuit.
  4–7 correct: Power surge.

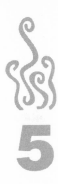

THE MENOPAUSAL BODY:

Livin' Large

Let's get ready to rummmmmmmble. . . . But first, we'll have to put on our size XL trunks. During menopause, I wasn't just fighting my husband, I was also fighting my weight. I mean, I wanted to be in shape, but not the oval shape I was in. What's worse, I was living in the most body-conscious era of all time. There's no escaping it. There are new gyms popping up next to the Starbucks on every corner all over town. I guess this explains why the entire population is awake all night exercising.

The truth is that after menopause, my body went downhill faster than Picabo Street on a black slope in Aspen. I had a lot of new stuff to contend with, because of my dwindling hormones. Sometimes I think it would be easier to be a man. But then, I don't really believe any of those lame theories proposed by Freud. Especially the one about penis envy. Hellooooo. There's no way I'd want to have a penis. My pants are already tight enough as it is.

Thin and Thinner

The number one goal of American women is to lose weight. Many women are literally killing themselves to be skinny. What's worse, this whole weight mania is continually fueled by the media. Every time I pick up a magazine or turn on the TV, I see supermodels who have less meat on them than a Slim Jim.

Just look at the current teen idols, like the pop singer Christina Aguilera. Or what about TV stars like Callista Flockhart and Lara Flynn Boyle? These gals must subsist on a diet of sprouts and crabgrass. Talk about your sixty-pound weaklings. There's no way you'll ever see one of these ladies pumping iron in a gym. These girls must have trouble lifting a number 2 lead pencil. The really sad thing is that too many women buy into this unrealistic image, and develop eating disorders trying to achieve it.

When I was a teenager, who knew from eating disorders? Clothes in size 2 and 3 didn't even exist. We all wore those "chubbette" sizes, and were totally happy with the way we looked. No starving ourselves, no neuroses. You might say, we lived large and loved it.

But nowadays you not only have to be thin, you have to be thin *and* toned. That's why memberships at fitness centers and spas are at an all-time high. But, here's the thing. They'll tell you anything to get you to join. But once they've got you, don't kid yourselves. They don't sit around and flatter you all day. When I first joined my gym, I took high-impact classes, where they totally kicked your butt for an hour. And when I got winded and started slacking a little, the instructor would always spot me among thirty other students and yell at me. I felt like boot camp might be easier. They won't let you keep your middle-aged flab. It's like, once you go through the door, they immediately sic trainers on you who run around with fat calibraters. They clamp those things onto your cellulite, and give you a readout. Then they mercilessly deliver the news* that your body is composed of 80 percent fat.

* Over the public address system.

In my case, all the buffed and toned members recoiled in horror. To them, this number was more humiliating than scoring in the 20th percentile on the SATs. I wasn't going to be able to look at myself* until I reached that target 6 percent.

Bathing Suit Blues

T. S. Eliot had it right when he said April was the cruelest month. That's because it's the month when I start shopping for a bathing suit. I like winter, because I can hide my body under sweat suits. I don't ever take a peek to see what I've morphed into. But as summer approaches, I've got no choice—unless I can find a bathing suit with long sleeves and feet.

To me, trying on a bathing suit in a department-store dressing room qualifies as a near-death experience. It's always a shock to look at my body after it's been in hibernation for months. Even worse, I have to look at it in those unflattering mirrors under their horrendous lighting. Can't they do anything to soften the blow? Like twenty-watt soft-glow bulbs or frosted mirrors? Give me a break. What I witnessed was more shocking than Hugh Rodham in a thong.

The salesgirls are also way out of touch with reality. For openers, they're all nineteen years old and wear size 2. They keep coming in with these teeny-weeny bikinis that have less material than Letterman on Monday nights. These new bathing suits are a cruel joke. They bare everything and cover nothing. The leg holes are slit clear up to the crests of my hips, my butt cheeks hang out, and the tops are nothing more than a pair of pasties connected by a string.

Whatever happened to that old one-piece number with the pleated skirt and built-in Tupperware bra? That baby could hide saddlebags bigger than Trigger's. Now, there was a suit that was flattering for women of all sizes. Unfortunately, the last time I saw one of them, it was on Marion Ross at a *Happy Days* reunion.

* More correctly—my butt.

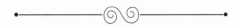

But Seriously . . .

If It Grows, Eat It

After menopause, our metabolism slows down. The reality is that we're going to gain weight more easily. So in order to keep our weight under control, we're going to need to start exercising in addition to watching what we eat.

I didn't go on a weight-loss diet, but I did change *what* I ate. Now I eat grilled fish, fresh veggies, and fruit with honey when I crave sweets. I avoid anything processed. I try to eat only that which comes from nature. I exercise six days a week. Here's the proof of the pudding. Now fifty-seven, I am 5'6", weigh 122 pounds, and wear a size 6. My cholesterol is 155 and my blood pressure is 110/70. I look and feel great.

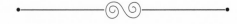

Waxing

When I tried on a bikini bottom, that was another terrible shock. When I saw myself in the mirror, at first I thought I was standing behind a shag rug. But on closer inspection, I realized it was just me—in dire need of a bikini wax.

Did you ever have one of these done? No? Well, here's my advice. Have a few Percodan and get your morphine IV drip ready. Mercy! We're talking major pain here. First off, the aesthetician* poured hot wax all over my most tender parts. Then she applied a waxing strip. After the wax cooled, she tore the strip off, ripping the hair out by the roots. What a jolt! Now I know what those guys on death row in Texas go through.

The good news is that after menopause, the situation gets

* Graduate of the Mengele Institute.

better. One result of decreasing estrogen levels is less body hair. At least that's an upside. Before menopause, I was like an ape. I had to get waxed at least every two weeks. And when I was through, they could have knitted scarves for the entire Russian army. It's a comforting thought to know that after menopause, the only waxing I'll have to do is on my car.

Liposuction

This is a perfect solution for women who just can't face those grueling workouts at the gym. There are women who have no idea whatsoever what their lats and quads are—much less how to target them. But as they say, everything has it's price. So don't be fooled into thinking that liposuction is going to be a walk in the park. Think New York Marathon in 100 percent humidity and you've got it.

Liposuction is touted as another one of those "simple and painless" cosmetic procedures. Excuse me. I don't think so. Being knocked out cold under a general anesthetic and sucked with a hose is anything but. The only person that this procedure is simple and painless for is the surgeon.

My girlfriend Sally told me the worst part of liposuction isn't the actual surgery. It's getting prepped. That's the part where they made her stand there naked while they circled all her fat pouches with a giant red Magic Marker. Yep, you heard me right. Her lumps and bumps were mapped out like a giant AAA Trip-Tik. She said it was so humiliating, she actually looked forward to the anesthesia.

You don't want to be awake for this operation—trust me. The surgery can take up to a few hours. It depends on how many Twinkies and DoveBars passed through your lips and were deposited directly on your thighs. The surgeon uses an instrument called a cannula to suck out all of your fat cells. It's such a nasty procedure, there's less blood and violence during three continuous showings of *Gladiator*. Sally sent her anesthesiologist a fruit basket to show her gratitude.

Remember, this procedure is not to be used in place of diet

and exercise. But when it's done in moderation, the results are usually excellent. The good news is that after a week's recovery period, Sally *felt* like her old self again. The bad news is that if she gains any new weight, she'll *look* like her old self again.

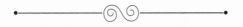

But Seriously...

Liposuction Lowdown

Although I have never had this procedure done, I do know one point that is very important: There are doctors licensed to perform liposuction who are not cosmetic surgeons. Any physician in any specialty who completes the required courses can obtain a license to do liposuction. Besides their regular practice, some doctors perform liposuction for extra income.

Be very careful to check the credentials of any doctor performing this procedure. Way too many deaths are reported as a result of liposuction because a doctor has removed too much body fat at one time. As with everything else, research your doctor and the procedure before having it done. This procedure is not to be dismissed as minor surgery. There is pain from liposuction and a decent recovery period is required.

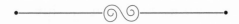

Abdominal Surgery

Because liposuction isn't always permanent, many women go for the more dramatic tummy tuck. But be warned: Even though it has a cutesy little name, it's anything but cute. This is a major surgical procedure. The surgeon cuts into the belly muscles, removes fat and other tissue, and then sews the abdominal muscles back together. The results are amazing, though. It's really impressive how flat and tight the abdomen looks.

A tummy tuck is a lengthy operation—it takes several hours—and it has a lengthy recovery time, too. How long? Let's just say that if you have it done when your kids are little, plan on being in the recovery room until their high school graduation. Okay, I exaggerated. Until junior high.

Mirror, Mirror on the Wall

I don't know. Isn't there an easier way to look thinner without all the pain and risk? We'd be better off creating an optical illusion to make ourselves appear skinny. Here are some tricks of the trade that have a long and glorious history—and they still work:

Oldies but Goodies

Big hair. Remember the old "Texas tease" that was popular back in the sixties? You know the style I'm talking about. The hairdo that looked like you were wearing a helmet? This coif was teased and sprayed until it became totally immobile. Just like a TV anchorperson's. Don't laugh. I've got news for you. There still are a lot of women who wear this style. That's because no matter how much weight they gain, an inflated head makes their bodies look small in comparison.

The women in the South have been wearing this style for so long, it's become part of their culture. For them, it's actually a religious experience. The bigger the hair, the closer to God.

Shoulder pads. Big shoulders create the illusion of a tiny waist and slim hips. That's why women have always loved the wide-shouldered look. It's always in fashion. You can get it by wearing shoulder pads in all sizes. The huge ones that look like you're wearing pillows on your shoulders are the best, though.

Remember Joan Crawford? She was the queen of the shoulder pads. Watching her old movies, you can see that no matter how big she got, her shoulder pads got even bigger. When her weight hit 165 pounds, she began wearing her suits with the hangers still in them. She even wore them to bed. In fact, the only time she removed them was when she wanted to punish her kids.

Caftans. Many of the aging stars, like Liz Taylor, favor these instead of clingy gowns. As they get older and pack on the pounds, these billowy garments become a staple in their wardrobes.

They can still look glamorous and hide a lot of weight at the same time. Many caftans are low-cut, so they still can be sexy. And a woman doesn't have to wear an uncomfortable strapless bra, either. She can show a lot of cleavage by hoisting up her ample bosoms with duct tape. Not only that, but she can install a heating or cooling system under there, too, for year-round comfort.

Collagen injections. These same women go overboard on the full, pouty lips. Remember Goldie Hawn's in *The First Wives Club*? Many women feel that oversized lips make their faces look much thinner.

But collagen injections can be expensive and painful, and the procedure is not without side effects. I find that I can get the same look by zipping up a pair of size 6 jeans until my lips swell.

Herbal wrap. This treatment will cost you big bucks at a fancy spa. Basically, they smear your naked body in gooey mud and herbs, then wrap you tightly in cellophane. They claim you not only shed a few pounds, but can lose up to two inches around your thighs, midriff, and upper arms.

Let's see. Gooey stuff . . . Saran Wrap . . . Haven't we heard this somewhere before? Oh, yeah. The writer Marabel Morgan, a maven on man-snagging and -enslaving advice, used to wrap herself up this way and greet her husband at the front door every night. She claimed that it turned him on and kept him coming home to her. I must admit, she got results. Just not the ones she had in mind. The good news: She lost over a hundred pounds. The bad news: It was her husband.

Gravity machine. With this piece of exercise equipment you are suspended upside down, with your feet in a pair of secured boots. You can hang there, say, in a doorway, for varying amounts of time. It's a form of passive exercise that is supposed to redistribute your weight and improve your circulation. But don't expect miracles. It won't turn a 32-28-38 body into a 38-28-32, no matter how long you hang there.

It takes a lot of guts* to get through a life passage like menopause. It also takes a sense of humor. But at least we have options. We can choose to age gracefully or fight back, like consumer advocate David Horowitz. One thing is for sure. The menopausal body needs more daily maintenance than one of Burt Reynolds's toupées. Maybe the best thing is to do nothing. Many feminists have been telling us all along to celebrate our wrinkles and gray hair.

I have given it a lot of thought, and decided to let nature take its course. I will not have surgery or lose weight just to look younger and thinner. That's just too egotistical. Me? I've decided to take the high road. I'm going to start hanging out with a bunch of overweight seventy-year-olds.

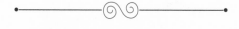

But Seriously . . .

When Fat Is Good

Though my cancer treatment ultimately didn't include chemotherapy, my doctor and I discussed the possibility. She stressed that I would need to maintain a high-fat diet prior to and after chemo, because chemo destroys healthy tissue along with the cancerous tissue and my body would need all the available resources it could get to quickly rebuild that tissue. That's why, if you are undergoing chemotherapy, weight gain is desirable. You can always lose the extra weight later.

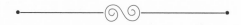

* But watch out—too much gut is a bad thing.

·Quiz·

Here's Looking at You, Kid

1. Jack Nicholson lost the sixty pounds he gained during midlife by . . .
   a. working out
   b. going on the Jenny Craig diet
   c. fasting twice a week
   d. breaking up with Lara Flynn Boyle

2. The part of you that most frequently gets bruised in the gym is your . . .
   a. shins
   b. calf muscles
   c. tendons
   d. ego

3. It might be a good time to lose weight when your photos . . .
   a. make you unhappy
   b. make you look ten pounds heavier
   c. need air-brushing
   d. have to be taken by satellite

4. Liposuction is recommended for your thighs when you walk and . . .
   a. your thighs jiggle
   b. you develop muscle cramps
   c. you get winded
   d. your pants burst into flame

5. When you go shopping for a bathing suit, it's best to prepare yourself by . . .
   a. dieting for two weeks
   b. working out for a month
   c. wearing a girdle
   d. wearing blinders
6. Women going through menopause should stay away from . . .
   a. salt
   b. alcohol
   c. sugar
   d. miniskirts

7. One sign of an aging body is when your gynecologist examines you . . .
   a. and prescribes hormones
   b. for decreasing estrogen
   c. more thoroughly
   d. wearing a hard hat

Quiz Results

The answers to all of the above are d, as in "Dexatrim."

   1–3 correct: You need to target your abs.

   4–7 correct: You need to shop at Target.

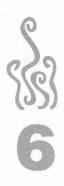

6

COSMETIC SURGERY:

Need a Lift?

Menopause isn't so bad if you think of it as a new frontier. You know—like the Space Age. It's a perfect analogy, because our bodies are falling faster than the Mir space station. Gravity happens. It's a real downer. So from now on, we'll be spending all our time and money pulling everything up.

Eyelids droop, jowls happen, and the phrase "turkey neck" suddenly is on everyone's lips. It's like one day we look in the mirror and see our mothers staring back at us. But we'll need to squint, because our vision is going, too. Like Electra, we're in a state of perpetual mourning. But in our case, it's not all that becoming.

My girlfriends tell me not to sweat it—I look great for my age. I'm healthy, have a good husband—blah, blah, blah. Yeah, I know all about it. I've heard it all before. The feminists say we should be proud of a face that's etched with character. Fine. But does my character have to look like Howdy Doody?

A Stitch in Time

I've tried the face exercisers, the creams, and the collagen. Now I'm afraid the only lasting solution is a face-lift. But the prospect scares me more than Anna Nicole Smith in a push-up bra. Did you ever take a good look at those aging stars on Academy Awards night? Never have so many been pulled so tight. These women have had their faces pulled up more times than Ted Kennedy's pants. Give me a break. When they chew, their eyebrows go up and down.

But no matter how opposed I had been to looking like a wax figure from Madame Tussaud's, when I turned fifty-seven, I caved in. Actually, my face did first. That's what sent me to a plastic surgeon for a consultation. I learned a lot. Believe me, it was a real eye opener.* So, now's your time to step up to the plate and take advantage of my experience. It's your opportunity to live vicariously through me. I'm going to tell you exactly what to expect when you decide to have a face-lift.

The lingo. It is not politically correct to call it "plastic surgery" anymore. Well, excuuuuse me. The doctors now refer to themselves as "cosmetic surgeons." Remember that. If you slip up and call one a plastic surgeon, it'll make his or her stethoscope curl. Not only that, but he or she will probably charge you double.

The whole practice of cosmetic surgery is based on politically correct language. The doctors are experts not only at reconstruction with the knife, but at reconstructing unacceptable words and ideas as well.

The office. When I walked into the surgeon's office, all I could think of was one of the designer rooms pictured in *Architectural Digest.* It was decorated in expensive fabrics from top-of-the-line companies such as Scalamandré and Brunswig & Fils, which positively scream old money. The furnishings were Louis XIV or XV—whichever year featured the most silk tassels and gilded trimmings.

---

* Before and after the blepharoplasty.

I was ushered into the salon area and invited to sit on a buttery-soft, leather sofa. Gazing around, I recognized the Mario Buatta chintz draperies and Tabriz Persian throw rugs. There were signed oil paintings and numbered lithographs on the walls. Not a hint of Holiday Inn to be found. In fact, if a polyester fiber happened to find its way onto the premises, they would immediately call in an exterminator.

The surgeon. My surgeon was the total embodiment of the look he was selling. Tanning-booth perfect, his handsome face was tight and unlined. He also was in possession of a fabulous cleft chin, which I'm sure he fashioned himself.

Gracing his mahogany desk were framed pictures of his gorgeous-looking family. Everybody was a perfect 10. Even the dog had capped teeth.

The consultation. For the purposes of maintaining anonymity and avoiding a potential lawsuit, I will call my surgeon Dr. Philip Flawless. Dr. Flawless had his Stepford staff take pictures of my face from every conceivable angle. Twenty minutes later, Dr. Flawless came back with my photos and a more carefully contrived speech than the one Bill Clinton gave the nation when he tried to explain away the Cuban cigar incident.

Cosmetic surgeons not only hold diplomas from the American College of Surgeons, but also hold degrees from the Emily Post School of Extreme Diplomacy. Dr. Flawless carefully chose words of the most nonoffensive nature possible. The guy was so good, he could mediate for disgruntled postal workers.*

The fees. A word of caution: You must never mention the words "Medicare" or "insurance coverage" to cosmetic surgeons. They make them nauseated.

All the distasteful talk about charges and fees was handled by his discreet office manager, Miss Moneypenny. I was ushered into the financial consultation room, which was yet another living tribute to Sister Parrish. The room also had another nice touch, silk moiré padded walls. Decorative? Yes. But their real

* Armed with AK-47's.

function was to muffle the screams when Moneypenny informs the patient how much it's going to cost.

But rest assured, it's money well spent. Dr. Flawless's patients come out looking gorgeous. He is always happy with his work. His wife is even happier, because she'll be wrapping her buffed butt in another fur coat. The money is also going for another worthy cause, education. His kids are happy because they won't have to be seen in the most unmentionable politically incorrect place of all—public school.

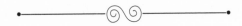

But Seriously...

It'll Cost You

Face-lifts have come a long way in the past few years. Many cosmetic surgeons use microsurgical incisions, lasers, and laparascopes to get a better result less invasively. You can opt to have remedial work done on just your eyes, your jowls and neck, or your forehead—or any combination of the three.

Yes, they are expensive. Out here in L.A., you've got to figure on around $15,000 to $20,000 for the whole megillah. Sure, there are some doctors who are cheaper, but as with any medical procedure, I feel that this is *not* the place to go bargain hunting. Unfortunately, often the old adage holds true: You get what you pay for.

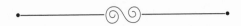

What he said. Dr. Flawless said I had a few "problem areas" that needed correction. He chose his words impeccably. Saggy areas were called "redundant skin". Wrinkles were "anatomical folds." Not once did the word "fat," "jowls," "bags," "sags," or "wrinkles" pass through his surgically sculpted lips.

What he thought. "Who the hell does she think I am—David Copperfield? The woman's got the jowls of J. Edgar Hoover and more wrinkles than my shar-pei. It's going to take me eight hours and a hundred yards of steel suture to haul that mess up and attach it. I wonder if I can do it without making her look like the Bride of Frankenstein. I'll be lucky if she isn't talking through her belly button for the rest of her life."

What I heard. "Jan, you're a wonderful candidate for cosmetic surgery. I will be lifting this redundant skin around your jawline, and pulling it back through tiny incisions behind your ears. I will lift the skin on your forehead, removing all the mature sections. The incision will be concealed in your hairline. The skin around your eyes will be tightened and smoothed.

"The result will be a youthful, rested look—not pulled and tight. It will take ten years off your appearance."

What I knew. I've seen many of my girlfriends immediately after their face-lifts. And believe me, I took one look at them and had to stifle a scream. They looked as though they had been assaulted with a baseball bat. Think Genghis Khan on steroids. All I could see was a giant head that looked as though it might explode any second.

However, they said there was no real pain, just discomfort. Uh-oh. There's that word again. Translation: They're within three seconds of losing control and screaming their swollen heads off. I'd say that was about a 50 mg Percodan tablet worth of discomfort.

The recuperation. I was given a list of things *not* to do after surgery:

No smoking

No drinking

No sun

No late hours

This means that even though I would look absolutely smashing, I'd be dull as dishwater. Oh, well. At least I'd be a youthful, unlined, unwrinkled bore while recuperating in cosmetic hell.

The debate. The one thing I had to ask myself was, "Is all this necessary?" Can't I go gently into that good night as I am—

without the nips, tucks, and lifts? And once I undergo one surgical procedure, will it ever end? The surgeons push it. They're always urging you to have another procedure done to correct every new line and wrinkle.

I'll tell you one thing. If I ever become one of those surgery junkies who has her parts recycled more often than her trash, somebody had better take me out with a laser.

I say this because I have a girlfriend who got caught up in this vicious cycle. In her case it was inevitable, because she was married to a cosmetic surgeon. She had him do twenty procedures in twelve years on her face and body—from cheek implants to liposuction. She had so much done over the years that even her dog didn't recognize her. But sadly, she and the surgeon husband eventually divorced. I guess there was nothing left to lift.

The good news is, we have some wonderful menopausal role models to follow in this millennium. They are women who have shown us that you can have a successful career that isn't beauty- or age-dependent.

Look at Gloria Steinem. An editor, feminist, and total babe in her sixties. Joan Rivers started a jewelry empire in her fifties. Liz Taylor went from being perhaps the silver screen's greatest star to being one of the most influential AIDS fund-raisers in the country. Farrah Fawcett celebrated fifty by dipping her naked body in paint and rolling around on a canvas, creating body art. She also gave a few memorable TV interviews that were completely incomprehensible to the human mind. Jane Fonda dumped her mogul hubby, Ted, at sixty-four. And Zsa Zsa slugged her first cop at seventy. You go, girls!

I'd say these gals deserve a big cheer. Some of these women have had cosmetic work and some haven't. The point is that we are all free to choose what's best for us. Go ahead. Throw in a face-lift if it floats your boat. You can sail around Golden Pond any way you choose. Don't feel guilty. Have it done as often as you want. It's always a good idea to put your best face forward—even if it is a different one every year.

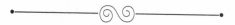

But Seriously...

For Best Results

A big factor in the success of your cosmetic surgery will be how well you follow doctor's orders. It's imperative that you do exactly what he or she tells you. No aspirin or vitamin E prior to surgery (slows down blood clotting) and no sun and no strenuous activity for a month following surgery. And most important of all—*no smoking!*

Smokers don't heal as well as nonsmokers, and their wrinkles come back a whole lot quicker. So if you're a smoker contemplating cosmetic surgery, it's best to quit before you have it. In fact, there are doctors who won't operate on smokers because their results aren't nearly as good as with nonsmokers.

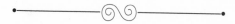

Sorry. You can't relax just yet. I'm not through with our body check. Groan. All this discussion about sagging reminds me of what I wanted to talk about in the first place. Boobs. Or, more accurately, menopausal boobs. I mean, just look in the mirror. Talk about going south. Those perky little mountains have become flatter than the state of Florida. Nowadays, I need a lot more than a padded bra. I need some oomph.

Making Mountains out of Molehills

There are several ways to add oomph to your chest. Basically, they fall into two categories: surgical and nonsurgical. Not all of them are completely safe, either. For example, one method is silicone implants. We are all aware that there are some serious health issues associated with silicone breast implants. However,

I'm not going to talk about them here. I'm going to leave that for Erin Brockovich to investigate. I'm just going to tell you what I know from personal experience.

The fact is that many women define their entire self-image by the size and shape of their breasts. How many times have you heard a woman say that she wants to have implants because large breasts will give her "confidence"? That they will raise her "self-esteem"? They will give her a feeling that she can "conquer the world"? Oh, shut up. They're boobs, for God's sake—not motivational speakers.

We have always been obsessed about breast size in this country. Both men and women spend a good part of their lives having intellectual discussions about whether certain celebrities have or haven't had boob jobs. For three years now, there has been an ongoing debate as to whether Britney Spears's are real or fake. The media coverage of Britney's boobs even takes precedence over the latest war in the Middle East. I'd say this is a pretty good indication that as a nation, we have way too much time on our hands.

This issue will probably be settled one day when we open the morning paper and read the headline: BRITNEY'S BREASTS RECALLED BY FIRESTONE.

Hey, I'm not exaggerating. Out here in L.A., breast implants aren't just a matter of personal choice—they're the law. And the bigger the better. Women have to compete with the likes of Pamela Anderson, Carmen Elektra, and Susan Sarandon. Over 90 percent of the world's mammary tissue is located right here in Hollywood. The women in L.A. have their breasts made so huge, they need to get a building permit before surgery.

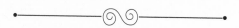

But Seriously...

Rearranging Priorities

After I was diagnosed with breast cancer, the thing I was most concerned about was saving my life. I would do whatever it took. I had always had a youthful bustline and wore clingy and moderately sexy clothing. But that didn't matter to me anymore. Preserving my life was a lot more important than having a sexy bustline. I was shocked when my doctor told me that even today, some of his patients say they would rather die than lose their breasts. I think that we women need to reevaluate our priorities about the importance of our breasts in our lives. If women truly believe their breasts are more important than life itself, something is terribly wrong.

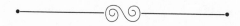

Surgical Approach

Don't get me wrong. Any woman who wants to get breast implants should do it. What gets me, though, is the rhetoric surrounding the decision. I am so tired of hearing women say that they want implants just to make themselves happy. What a crock. Did you ever see one of these gals get those double-D knockers and then hide them under a baggy sweatshirt? No way. At $5,000 each, you can be sure they're going to be hanging out of a décolletage, right in everyone's face.

Here's another one of my juicy true stories. This one is about how my girlfriend publicly debuted her implants.

My husband and I had dinner with our friends Heather and Gregg. Heather is fortyish, and a natural knockout to begin with. But that evening, I couldn't take my eyes off her. Correction: her chest. Her breasts were so inflated, they were resting on the table. Likewise, her sweater was stretched to the maximum safety point recommended by the Lycra company before the fiber spontaneously explodes. In fact, I couldn't tell you about anything we had for dinner, because I couldn't take my eyes off those mammoth creatures. She didn't just look like a waitress from Hooters, she looked like the whole franchise.

Heather whispered in my ear, "Jan, do you notice anything *different* about me?"

How do you answer this? "I sure do. I notice that your breasts need their own zip codes."

Instead, I say the polite thing. "Not really—other than that you look gorgeous, as usual."

"Well, I just had a nipple lift," she confided.

"Come again?" I said, coughing and spewing out half of my piña colada.

"A nipple lift. It's when the surgeon adds some implants on the side of your breasts, then lifts them up so they look perkier."

"Well, they certainly do look very, very perky," I said emphatically.

"I just love the look. It makes me feel so great about my body. And my husband can't keep his hands off me."

"A fantasy every man in this restaurant shares," I said with a big grin.

During our conversation, I'm thinking that now I've heard and seen everything. A *nipple* lift? It must be for depressed boobs. "Do boobs get depressed?" I wonder. "And if so, why not put them on Prozac, like everybody else?" Give me a break! I feel like the whole female population around me is going nuts. I could fill a phone book with the names of friends who have had tummy tucks, breast implants, face-lifts, liposuction—and now "nipple lift" is added to the list. Whatever happened to the old padded bra? I guess it's in the Smithsonian along with Carol Channing's eyelashes.

I knew I shouldn't put my husband on the spot, but I couldn't stop myself. I had to ask him what he thought about Heather and her magnificent melons. So on the way home, I popped the "big one."

"So—what do you think of Heather's new friends?"

"What are you talking about, Jan?" he asked warily.

"Now, don't get all coy on me. You *had* to notice the additional sixty pounds of mammary tissue resting on our table this evening."

"Oh—those," he said, laughing. "What do you think?"

"Stop playing psychiatrist with me and tell me what *you* think," I pressed on.

"You won't get mad?"

"Of course not. Just tell me."

"I think they're pretty sexy. She has the body to carry them off very nicely."

"Well, maybe I should consider having mine done, too," I said petulantly.

Rule 1: Never believe a woman who says she won't get mad at the truth.

"Over my dead body," he replied.

"Oh, I get it," I said sarcastically. "It's okay for Heather to have a sexy body, but I should wear my AAA-cup training bra for the rest of my life?"

"Don't be ridiculous, Jan. You are the sexiest woman I know, with the best set of hooters in town."

"Gee, thanks, honey."

Rule 2: Quit while you're ahead!

End of discussion. The man had obviously studied with the master—Dr. Phil Flawless.

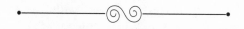

But Seriously . . .

The Nipples Cost Extra!

Many women are not aware that when a mastectomy is performed, the surgeon removes your nipple. That's because nipples contain millions of tiny ducts where cancer cells may hide out. Fortunately, the surgeon can reconstruct a nipple a few months after the mastectomy. Either he or she creates a new nipple from your own breast skin or uses skin grafted from your inner thigh or vagina. The total cost of this surgery is $1,000 to $1,500. A few months after constructing my nipples, my surgeon tattooed areolas around them. They are lighter in color than my originals, but they look really pretty—kinda like a Barbie doll's.

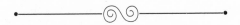

Nonsurgical Approach

For women who are opposed to surgery, there are other ways of achieving that full-busted look.

The Wonderbra. Nowadays, we have the technology to make mountains out of molehills without surgery. The Wonderbra revolutionized this arena. It works like magic. Even David Copperfield can't figure out how Claudia does it. In fact, the Wonderbra should use the slogan "Presto! Breasto!"

With its ingenious use of underwire and padding on the sides of the cups, it does the impossible. It could even give cleavage to Dennis Rodman.

Liquid-filled Miracle Bra. This ingenious bra boosts the bust with liquid-filled pads. The bust not only looks natural but feels natural, too. The real beauty of a water bra is that it doesn't pose any health risks to the person wearing it. It's actually a bit protective. The only bruise you might get while wearing one is to your ego—if you spring a leak in public.

Duct tape. With today's revealing décolletages and backless numbers, we have to be resourceful. That's why women are flocking to Home Depot to purchase the latest trend in underwear: duct tape.

Remember J.Lo's famous dress she wore to the Grammys? *Va-va-voom.* It was miraculous how she kept anything hidden under so little material. We may never be sure how she did it. But one thing we can be sure of is that she was not carrying any concealed weapons.

Tissue. An oldie but a goodie. I started stuffing tissue in my bras during junior high. Whether I stuffed a few or a whole bunch, nobody ever knew. And if any of them unexpectedly popped out of my strapless, I'd always use the same old alibi—chest cold.

Now, wasn't this chapter uplifting? Even if we are losing the war against poverty and drugs, it's comforting to know that we are winning the war against gravity.

· Quiz ·

Test Your Surgical Savvy

1. After multiple cosmetic surgeries, Michael Jackson looks like . . .
   a. he's twenty years old
   b. a different person
   c. his younger sister
   d. his negatives

2. You should consider a face-lift when you have to airbrush your photos . . .
   a. to remove unsightly wrinkles
   b. to look as you did in your thirties
   c. with professional equipment
   d. with a caulking gun

3. It's time for a face-lift when you are applying your makeup . . .
   a. with a sponge
   b. for over an hour
   c. with a magnifying mirror
   d. using a paint-by-numbers set

4. The most common cause of premature wrinkles is . . .
   a. smoking
   b. the sun
   c. alcohol
   d. your kids

5. Post-op sedation should only be necessary . . .
   a. in a very few cases
   b. when the patient can't sleep
   c. during the removal of stitches
   d. when you open your bill

6. After a face-lift, most women have the facial expression of . . .
   a. a babe in the woods
   b. Botticelli's Venus
   c. a diva in the spotlight
   d. a deer caught in headlights

7. In Los Angeles, a death occurring during cosmetic surgery is ruled as . . .
   a. a homicide
   b. manslaughter
   c. an accident
   d. natural causes

8. Which celebrity popularized the strapless bra?
   a. Marilyn Monroe
   b. Jayne Mansfield
   c. Elizabeth Taylor
   d. David Bowie

9. In which movie did Madonna debut her bullet bra?
   a. *Desperately Seeking Susan*
   b. *Truth or Dare*
   c. *Body Heat*
   d. *Lethal Weapon 2*

10. What posed the most serious environmental threat on *Baywatch*?
    a. skin cancer from sun exposure
    b. littering by the film crew
    c. vandalism
    d. a major silicone spill

Quiz Results

The answers to all of the above are d, as in "dermabrasion."
   1–5 correct: It's not funny.
   6–10 correct: You're in stitches.

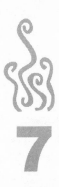

7

MALE MENOPAUSE:

Men Behaving Badly

Okay. Whaddya say? It's high time for some male bashing. So, open your dictionaries, please. Here's the deal. Way before *Webster's* was published, women always maintained that all our ailments began with "men." Now, it's official. Here are just a few in the very long list:

Menstruation

Menorrhagia

Mental illness

Menopause

So there you have it. The proof is in the testosterone pudding. Of course, all men deny it. But we know that this is no linguistic coincidence.

It's a universal truth that men just can't stand to be outdone. So in their predictable pattern of one-upmanship, they have come up with a syndrome parallel to menopause and dubbed it "male menopause." However, there's all kinds of controversy about whether men actually experience it during midlife. Is it a bona fide affliction or merely "in their heads"? If you ask me, I'd say it's the latter. Why not? That's what they've always said about everything we women suffer with—from periods to paralysis.

Adult males pretty much keep an even testosterone level. They don't experience the wildly fluctuating hormone levels that women do during menopause. So what's their excuse? Is there an actual medical reason for acting like jerks when they hit midlife? Who knows? But judging from their loony antics during "male menopause," one fact cannot be denied. Men, as a species, need to be *medicated*.

I readily admit that during menopause I got bloated, weepy, and often added chocolate chips to my cheese omelets. But these symptoms are nothing in comparison to the stunts my husband pulled. And all males do the same things! It's as predictable as another Robert Downey Jr. drug bust. It's really easy to spot a man who is going through a midlife crisis. He stands out more than Dennis Rodman* at a little people's convention.

The first symptom of my husband's male menopause was an overwhelming need to still feel attractive to the opposite sex. This, by itself, I could handle. But the real problem started when he felt like he had to go out and prove it.

Like you, I have always accepted the fact that guys spend the greater part of their lives checking out and/or scratching their private parts. But during male menopause, he obsessed about his sexual prowess. The importance of being potent, if you will. He considers old guys, like Tony Randall and Anthony Quinn, who have fathered children in their eighties as heroes. But isn't it typical of men to just focus on the act and not the consequences of their actions? Women don't call these old guys heroes. We call them irresponsible. We need somebody who is going to be around afterward to help raise our children. Who wants a guy who is going to drop dead an hour after copulating?

During his menopause, my husband experienced an epiphany that caused a huge shift in his priorities. All of a sudden, these three fears ruled his life. They are, in order of importance,

* In drag.

1. Impotence
2. Aging
3. Death

It's no wonder Viagra has become the drug of choice for men like him. You can bet that guys who never sought medical treatment for anything, including decapitation, are now beating down their doctors' doors to get these pills. And even the recent revelation that Viagra might make you blind hasn't slowed down sales. In fact, they've skyrocketed. I guess men feel that the important thing is that they are able to perform—they could care less who it's with.

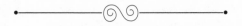

But Seriously . . .

Drawing the Line

Although they'll deny it to their deathbeds, I think that many men are just as concerned with physical aging as women are. When they start to act out, my advice is to give them some latitude. We all go a little nuts when confronting our mortality.

Nonetheless, behavior such as physical or verbal abuse, alcoholism, and infidelity shouldn't be viewed as acceptable midlife-crisis behavior. They are violations of your marriage vows and affronts to your dignity.

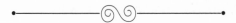

The irony is that my husband insists it's me who obsesses about getting older. Wrong. Who is he kidding? Getting older scares the pants off most men. Unfortunately, I mean this literally. Many good husbands fall victim to the *affaire du jour* in a misguided attempt to prove they are not only potent but also immortal. And they say women don't have a grasp on reality. At least we don't have delusions of being the freakin' Highlander on Viagra. Anyways, here are some of their class-action behaviors:

The Warning Signs

Buys a sports car. As long as there are middle-aged men in crisis out there, the sports-car manufacturers will never go under. My husband went through his own midlife crisis at fifty-three years of age. How did I know? He went out and bought a sports car. But not just any old garden variety of sports car. It was a superflashy late-model Corvette convertible in a shade of canary yellow that could be spotted from the space shuttle *Discovery*.

For some arcane reason, an open sports car has always been a symbol of sexual virility. Remember back in high school when a '63 Thunderbird convertible was considered a phallic symbol, and you were afraid to touch it? Well, times haven't changed that much. Forty years later, I still have to deal with my husband's adolescent thinking.

And speaking of Freudian symbols, how about this one? He insisted that the sports car must come with a stick shift. Give me a break. Do we need a visual here? In keeping with this phallic philosophy, he will probably order a hood ornament in the shape of a giant hot dog.

When he gets behind the wheel of that convertible, it makes him feel totally cool. I just don't get it. I hate having my hairdo blown to bits. He, on the other hand, loves the feeling of the wind gusting through his few remaining strands of hair. Or maybe it's the wind whistling through his nose after he removes the ring. Who knows? Who cares? But one thing is for sure. Men like their sports cars like their women—with the tops down.

Gets a trendy coif. Another sign of crisis was when my husband ditched "Little Joe," his barber of twenty years. He now feels it is incumbent upon him to go to a trendy "stylist" with a name like Claudio Issyake. "Stylist" translated from the Latin means "jacked-up price." The thing is, he always complained about the ten dollars he had to fork over to "Little Joe."* But

* Plus the fifty-cent tip.

now he's only too happy to write a check for $150 in an ego-stroking salon called Virility. Go figure.

For years, this man wore a low-maintenance crewcut with enough wax to turn the hair into kabob spears. But now he spends hours getting moussed, gelled, and blow-dried. And God forbid when Mr. Head and Shoulders starts losing his hair. He'll turn to his new best friends, Propecia and Rogaine. Worse yet, I wouldn't be surprised to find he's a card-carrying member of the Hair Club for Men. Just think of that big, wide forehead as the site of future transplants. Like Samson, he believes his manhood emanates from his hair transplants or toupee.

Buys a cool wardrobe. Most men continue to wear the same pants they wore in high school throughout most of their adult years—except they're a lot lower now. But when male menopause happens, those trousers become history. My husband went for a total wardrobe makeover, starting from the inside out.

His geeky, paisley boxer shorts are now just a memory. Wow—I remember those things. He made me not only iron them but starch them, too. Well, it looks like he's trading in the Niagra to make room for the Viagra. Now, he's stocking up on microfiber stretch bikinis in Day-Glo colors. Okay, I can live with that. It's a harmless way to express his manhood. But God help me when he starts buying the kind with the padded cup. That's one of the signs of the apocalypse.

His classic khaki pants and Nautica shirts have also sailed off into the sunset. Now, he's strutting his stuff in chichi Italian suits with the pant legs wide enough to double as Dennis Conner's mainsail.

His standard-issue black plastic eyeglass frames have also been chucked.* Now he's sporting cool Brad Pitt–type shades with a mirror finish. Sure, they look cool, but they should come with a warning label. Those teeny-weeny lenses are so highly reflective, if he stares at a woman under the hot sun for more than two minutes, she could burst into flames.

The final step was when he traded in his beat-up Nikes for

---

* Along with the tape on the nose bridge.

Gucci loafers. Naturally, he wears them without socks. So now we've got the Versace suit, the Vuarnet shades, and the Gucci loafers. When he adds the de rigueur ponytail, he will have made his ultimate fashion statement: "I look like a horse's ass." What a joke. He's spending a fortune on himself. At this point, he's got more invested in his wardrobe than in his IRA.

Takes up extreme sports. At one time my husband felt that living on the edge meant drinking milk one day past the expiration date on the carton. But not so anymore. When midlife approached, he bought into the guy philosophy of not feeling "alive" unless he's living on the edge. Like, the edge of insanity.

He became obsessed with grabbing all the gusto he could get. Personally, I blame this insanity on beer commercials, not his hormones. But one thing is for sure. He is no longer content to be a couch potato, yelling guy stuff like "Boo-ya" at the TV. He's got to be out there, cavorting like he's twenty years old again.

This means taking up extreme sports like snowboarding, bungee jumping, sky diving, and tae kwan do. He's enrolled himself in the local martial arts academy, convinced he's going to be the next Bruce Lee. Oh yeah, right. At his age, the only movie he could land a starring role in is *Swollen Prostate, Hidden Hernia.*

Meanwhile, I feel totally helpless. There's nothing I can do to change his behavior. All I can do is wait and worry, hoping this too shall pass. On second thought—ix-nay on the orry-way. There is something I can do. Double his life insurance policy. This taunting-death stuff only works if he's got more lives than Shirley MacLaine.

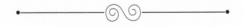

But Seriously ...

Guys: Not Perfect but Human

Don't expect your husband to be really sympathetic during menopause. Men just don't have the frame of reference to understand how difficult, physically and psychologically, menopause is for us. From my own experience, I found that a good sense of humor was the best tool in helping me cope with menopause and men.

It took my husband a while to become sensitive to my needs as I was struggling to cope with my new body after my mastectomies. Is he perfect? Nah. Sometimes he forgets and makes some dumb guy joke about fake boobs or breast-feeding. But so what? It's not that he doesn't love me. He's just being a guy. I've learned to relax and just go with that.

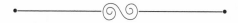

Frequents gentlemen's clubs. I was lucky that my husband didn't go this far. But during a midlife crisis many men decide that their homeboy haunts aren't going to cut it anymore. The old male-bonding stuff they once loved, like drinking, crushing beer cans on their heads, and watching beer shoot out of their noses just doesn't have the same magic. Now, they're into more "mature" pursuits. Uh-huh . . . "Mature pursuits" translated means watching boobs. They've discovered "classy" gentlemen's clubs. You know, strip joints with pretentious names like Rumours, Scores, and Scandals. So now he's chucked the beer-can crushing in favor of more lofty pursuits—like getting a lap dance.

Every middle-aged man feels it's his God-given right to experience a lap dance before he dies. Little does he know that it could happen at any moment, when some nineteen-year-old sticks her 42-DDD boobs into his face.

Just be on the alert. These behaviors will probably consume him for a few years. Be prepared for a husband who starts behaving like a six-year-old. It's going to be hard not to act like his mother instead of his wife. And when he hits the wall running, he will announce that he is "bored" and needs to "make some changes" in his life. Here's what my husband told me:

He needs space.

He needs to find himself.

He needs to explore his sexuality.

He needs to get in touch with his inner child.

During this period of infantile self-indulgence, I gave him a lot of love. Tough love. He wants space? Okey-dokey. Let him sleep in a big king-size bed—alone. He needs to find himself? Good. Dump him in the Everglades with a compass and a map. He wants to explore his sexuality? No problem. Send him to a local clinic for a sex lecture and a vasectomy. He wants to get in touch with his inner child? Easy. He can get in touch with a whole bunch of them when he drives the car pool for a month.

This plan took care of my male-menopause issue, ladies. It gave him more than a little taste of freedom—enough to choke on.

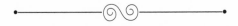

But Seriously ...

You're Never Too Old for Advice

The sad fact is that 50 percent of marriages end up in the divorce court. Many couples throw in the towel because they just can't talk to each other anymore. I ought to know. I've been married three times. But this time I did something different that has been invaluable to our marriage. I sought counseling when problems arose that I just couldn't handle myself. And when you're going through menopause, everyone around you is, too—believe me. Counseling can not only save marriages but make them stronger than ever.

Even though you're married, it doesn't mean that you stop growing and changing emotionally. Counseling gives you the opportunity to express both your positive and negative feelings in a safe environment. It leads to better communication, which allows you both to feel more secure in your marriage.

· Quiz ·

Bad Behavior

1. You find a bra and panties in the glove compartment of your husband's car. He claims . . .
   a. they're yours
   b. he has no idea how they got there
   c. he's sorry
   d. he's a cross-dresser

2. A middle-aged man's way of saying "You complete me" is with . . .
   a. flowers
   b. a romantic vacation
   c. a diamond ring
   d. a ménage à trois

3. During a midlife crisis, your husband will agree to counseling...
   a. if you attend with him
   b. only if it's an ultimatum
   c. on a trial basis
   d. with Charlie Sheen

4. During male menopause, a nonreligious man may turn to religion and emulate which leader?
   a. Gandhi
   b. Jerry Falwell
   c. Billy Graham
   d. Jesse Jackson

5. During a midlife crisis, many men begin riding their bikes every day because . . .
   a. it improves their cardiovascular system
   b. they want to lose weight
   c. it relieves stress
   d. they've had so many DUI's

6. Many overweight men find they can raise their heart rate most quickly with . . .
   a. the treadmill
   b. a three-mile run
   c. the StairMaster
   d. porno and cocaine

7. A man going through male menopause thinks that our number one national problem is the . . .
   a. unstable economy
   b. lowering of moral standards
   c. rising teenage pregnancy
   d. demise of Napster

Quiz Results

The answers to all of the above are d, as in "dirty rotten scoundrel."

1–3 correct: He's acting like a good daddy.

4–7 correct: He's acting like Puff Daddy.

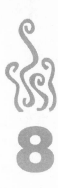

8

SEXUAL SATISFACTION:

An Oxymoron

There's no doubt about it. After menopause, my libido ended up in limbo. I don't think I actually lost it—I just misplaced it. How come? Is it a physical thing or a mental thing—or both? If you ask me, it's both. I and a million other menopausal women are plagued with low estrogen and high progesterone and suffer extreme emotional tension while counting our gray hairs and cellulite bumps. We're hot, we're cold, we're happy, we're sad—blah, blah, blah. Just give me a year of your time and I'd be delighted to tell you all about it.

My husband swears that the problem is all in our heads. What else did you expect him to say? Men are clueless about physical suffering. About the only thing he's ever suffered is a lot of gas. Even then, I end up the victim.

But one thing has been true since Eve experienced her first hot flash. Men have always complained they're not getting enough sex. No matter how frequently I give in to him, it's never enough. All I hear about is how "frigid" I am. He's always whining about this stuff—like his sex life has turned into thirty minutes of begging. Okay. So what's his point?

I don't have to tell you that there is a lot of controversy sur-rounding middle-aged sex. On one hand, there's the reality of what we are actually doing and on the other hand, what we are supposed to be doing. But I do know one thing. If I did every-thing that the dumb sex manuals suggest, I'd be in the ICU from any one of the following:

Exhaustion

Overexposure

Severe abrasions

Don't ask me about great menopausal sex. My husband is one of those men who subscribe to the theory that bad sex is better than no sex at all. He is always complaining that I'm never in the mood. In fact, just last night he said, "Honey, I can't remember the last time we had sex." So I said, "Oh, yeah? Well, I do. And that's why we're not doing it anymore."

But he kept complaining. He even went so far as to issue an ulti-matum. He said that because I am through menopause and the kids are gone, he is entitled to sex *twice a day,* not twice a week. Well, I've got news for him. As my husband, he is entitled to one of my kidneys and my bone marrow, but *this request* is out of the question.

Also, he can forget about phone sex, too. If I had to have any kind of sex twice a day, the only phone call I'd be making is to 911—for an ambulance. I've also told him never to wake me up at 6 A.M. to make love. Anybody who wakes me up for any rea-son before 9 A.M. gets one bullet in the head and two in the gut. Hey, so I'm not a morning person. You got a problem with that?

Passion Chart

In the lovemaking department, essentially this is what happens in the succeeding decades of life:

Twenties	**Thirties**	**Forties**	**Fifties**
Broad daylight on the beach	Nooner in the spa	Candlelit bedroom	In a room so dark, only bats can navigate it

I'll be the first to admit that after menopause, my sex life plummeted faster than the Tokyo stock exchange in 1998. The fact is that bodywise, after menopause I've got a lot more to hide. After having two kids, I developed stretch marks over 99 percent of my body. I am obsessed about finding the most flattering position to display my body during lovemaking. Let me tell you something. It's not an easy task.

Anyway, I have another valid excuse. You can't talk about a menopausal woman nowadays without mentioning three crucial words: "feminine moisture replacement."

It's an issue that's on the collective mind of all Americans. Just tune in to the six o'clock news and you'll hear Dan Rather and Tom Brokaw giving nightly reports about it. It's gotten so much national attention that Dick Cheney is heading up an ad hoc committee* to study the problem.

I don't care what my husband thinks. The need for feminine moisture replacement happens to be a very real phenomenon. He ought to try having sex with body parts drier than the Betty Ford Clinic. Whew. Forget the sex. Most days, it hurts just walking around. My gynecologist said that Astroglide would be a big help. But I hate those rides at Disneyland. Anyway, I don't see how that will help my problem.

---

* Which he is chairing from the ICU.

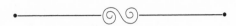

But Seriously . . .

Beefing Up the Libido

There is really no need to stress about a decreased libido after menopause, because this problem is totally normal. Dealing with vaginal dryness may improve sexual function. Ask your gynecologist about one of the new vaginal creams that supplies small doses of estrogen, which helps the tissue retain its natural moisture. The cream is absorbed topically, so it's even safe for breast cancer patients. If your libido could use a jump start, the male hormone testosterone is a big help. Doctors are prescribing it to many menopausal women these days. It's very safe, and according to several of my girlfriends, it *really works wonders.*

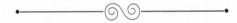

Marriage Manuals: Show-and-Tell

I may not be sexually dead after menopause, but I am in danger of dying of boredom. I'm definitely past the passion-filled years when I got drilled more often than Black & Decker. During menopause, I lost interest faster than one of Charles Keating's savings and loans. The trick was to find ways to perk up my interest and get myself back into the swing.* Sometimes, all it takes is a little imagination—and a lot of feminine-moisture-replacement products.

I bought some marriage manuals to see what kinds of activities they suggested. Mercy! Did you ever read one of these things? They've got to be kidding. Every other word is "hot:"

---

* Not the kind you hang from your ceiling.

"hot sex"; "hot foreplay"; "hot lips"; "hot blood." Is that so? Well, they don't have to tell me about being hot. During menopause, hot is all I ever felt. . . . Flashes, that is.

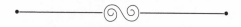

But Seriously . . .

Perking Up Takes Planning

My husband and I have found that if we take the time to plan a romantic getaway weekend, it does wonders to perk up our libidos. Because most couples are so engrossed in raising kids, doing well at work, and coping with daily struggles, they never find the time to be alone together. However, a little getaway or a standing date night does wonders to promote the feeling of still courting each other.

With a change of scene away from your home territory, you can actually hold an entire conversation without interruption. You have the time to bond again. The closeness you feel will naturally lead to great lovemaking. If you ask me, getting away is better than any kind of sexual pill on the market.

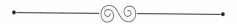

Here are some of the techniques the manuals suggest that promise guaranteed results:

The sensual bath. The "sensual bath experience" sets the stage for an erotic sexual encounter. The manual shows a sunken tub surrounded by dozens of glowing candles. They recommend scented candles, in all sizes and shapes. They're supposed to illuminate the room with soft, romantic light and fill it with heady, exotic smells. This looked pretty good to me, so I decided to try it.

But wouldn't you know it? I ran into a big problem. Four dozen burning candles give off a lot of smoke. Within minutes of luring my husband into the romantically illuminated "love tub," the smoke detector went off, ruining our chance for a "wet encounter" of *any kind.*

The oil and lube. Okay, so the sensual bath was a bust. But I wasn't going to get discouraged, so I switched to Plan B. In this exercise in erotic foreplay you massage each other with exotic love oils. I have to admit that my husband really got into it. The minute I began massaging him with the oils, his muscles relaxed. In fact, he relaxed so much, he was snoring within ten minutes. When I tried to wake him, he slid off the bed onto the floor. So I just left him there. Another romantic encounter gone wrong.

The next day, I was left with the distinctly unromantic task of laundering oily sheets. For all the results I got, I could have saved myself a few bucks by using Wesson oil. At least I could have fried up some chicken while he was unconscious.

The position statement. I'm not embarrassed to say it. In my younger days, I was a heck of a lot more adventurous about trying new sexual positions. Admit it. You were, too. We all kept a copy of the *Kama-Sutra* on our night tables for quick reference. In fact, after we mastered all the positions, we sent away for the supplement.

So what happened to us sexual athletes? Two words: muscle spasms. *Warning:* My husband and I got spasms in muscles we never knew we had. The manuals recommend that we should practice different positions regularly. Is that so? Well, here's my recommendation: Do them in total darkness, because all of these unusual positions are terribly unflattering to your menopausal body.

And while we're on the subject of unflattering positions, I'm never getting on top anymore. It makes me look like someone deflated my face. Also, any fooling around in a vertical position is out, too. The only thing I want to receive while standing is an ovation.

Even when we managed to execute one of the exotic positions, I didn't expect to get much out of it except a bad case of tendinitis. Which is what I got: I had to slather myself with smelly Ben-Gay, forcing my husband to sleep in the guest room all week. Uh-oh. Three for three. Looks like we're batting zero in the love games.

Toys for tarts. I don't think there's a snowball's chance in hell that someone could ever talk me into buying so-called love toys such as vibrators and French ticklers. Love toys just seem ridiculous to me. Maybe it's my Catholic upbringing. I don't know. But when it comes to this stuff, I'm more uptight than John Ashcroft at a Hooters convention.

Have you ever checked out the list of foods the love manuals suggest you add to sex? Whipped cream, honey, chocolate syrup—are you making love or a sundae? But the manuals don't stop there. The "toys" come in the later chapters, where they start pushing heavy-duty love accoutrements like handcuffs, studs, leather whips, and a whole array of battery-powered devices.

Not with me you don't. I'm not going down that road. My personal rule is that if it's a sexual activity involving anything edible, mechanical, or electrical, it's definitely not on my agenda. There is no power on earth persuasive enough to get me to use a vibrator with a battery large enough to start my car.

Academy Award–winning roles. I know role playing is very popular, but I just can't get into it. The thought of having to become someone else to get turned on really turns me off. The only time you'll find me in a costume is on Halloween. And even then I don't enjoy it. I'm in it strictly for the candy.

Every sex manual seems to push the "French maid" thing. Of course, it's great for men. My husband loves it when I'm in a servile position in the bedroom. Well, I've got news for him. I'm in servitude seven days a week as it is—without the mini-apron and push-up bra. At least give me a persona where I can exert some power—like Dominatrix Barbie.

However, I have to admit there was a brief period in my life when role playing worked really well for me. It was when I was pregnant. In my eighth month I played Mt. Everest, and my husband was Sir Edmund Hillary on a climbing expedition. Now, that was fun. It was kind of like the mile-high club without the costly airfare and the teeny bathroom. Then in my ninth month, when I morphed into a whale, I made a great Moby Dick to my husband's Captain Ahab. He spent hours trying to harpoon me. Welcome aboard, matey.

But other than those times, I say ix-nay on the sex role play. Being in drag is nothing but a drag.

The photo op. I'm going on record as stating that I am categorically opposed to any reproduction of my likeness during sex in the form of videos, Polaroids, or digitally reproduced photos. I look bad enough in my driver's license photo, so I can't imagine one of my entire body . . . naked.

What are you supposed to do with these photos, anyway? They're hardly suitable for a family album. Besides, how do you get up the nerve to face the guy at the Fotomat? Not to mention, once you have film of those incriminating shots, who knows what could happen? Like that poor Pamela Anderson. You must have read about that fiasco. Her love-romp videos ended up being sold all over the Internet. It was tragic. The woman was totally humiliated and outraged for obvious reasons: She never got to see a dime of the proceeds.

Call me old-fashioned, but I think that what we do in private should stay in private. Case in point: Tom Cruise and Nicole Kidman. After the public showing of their torrid love scenes in *Eyes Wide Shut,* the worst of all fates befell them—the movie bombed. Oh, yeah . . . they got divorced, too.

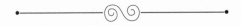

But Seriously . . .

Sex After Surgery

Many women fear that when they have a mastectomy and their nipple is removed, they will lose all sensation in their reconstructed breast (or breasts). They are afraid that the lack of breast sensation will put a real damper on their sex lives, especially their ability to achieve orgasm. Let me put your minds at rest. Yes, you will lose the sensation you once had in your nipples. But the breasts themselves regain most of their normal tactile sensation within the first year after surgery.

I found that my ability to experience an orgasm was even *better* after the surgery. Don't ask me why because I have no idea. Maybe it's the principle of a blind person developing a keener sense of hearing. Or maybe it's just that I have successfully learned to live in the moment. But whatever the reason, I consider it another gift along with my life.

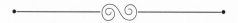

"True Lies." This brings me to another "kiss and tell" story featuring one of my girlfriends. By now, I know you're all thinking, "This woman just can't keep her mouth shut. How does she manage to keep any friends?" Easy. I always change the names to protect the guilty.

So here's the scoop on my girlfriend Molly. During a particularly vigorous night of lovemaking with her husband, she actually got her head caught between the slats of her headboard. The pain was so intense, she began shouting, "Ooh . . . ooh." But her husband mistook her cries as a rousing cheer for his bravura performance. This made him press on with even more gusto. She finally had to scream, "Stop it! Stop it!" before he realized it was not his male prowess that was driving her to wail so loudly.

It took her several minutes* to ease her head out from between the slats. But thank goodness she managed to do it without having to call for help. She had visions of being carried out of the house by the paramedics with her head still locked in the headboard-cum-vise. All the while, the gawking neighbors would rupture their spleens laughing.

Well, there you have it—another testament to testosterone.

---

* And a jar of Vaseline.

By the way, there's a lesson to be learned from this story. I'm not sure what it is, though. But I do know this: We gals should quit worrying about all this sex stuff. It really doesn't matter what we do, because there is no force on earth great enough to deflate the male ego. All we have to do is show up.

So, here's my review of love manuals. Most of their suggestions are either unsafe or just plain stupid. I have rejected the candle caper on the grounds that it might incinerate me. Massaging my husband with love oils made every muscle in my body stiff, while all of *his* went limp. You might say the whole experience was anticlimactic. The aerobic foreplay is definitely going to incapacitate me. And finally, I firmly believe that the only people who should be playing with battery-powered toys are my grandkids.

All this fooling around is just too dangerous. From now on, the only risks I'll be taking are in the stock market.

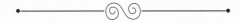

Sexual Savvy

Q: What do they call the skin around a penis?
A: A man.

Q: Why do men prefer virgins?
A: They can't take criticism.

Q: What is the difference between a husband and a lover?
A: Forty-five minutes.

Q: Why do women fake orgasms?
A: Because men fake foreplay.

Q: What's the name of the disease that paralyzes women from the waist down?
A: Marriage.

Q: What is the end result of penile enlargement?
A: Bigger prisons.

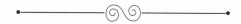

As if I didn't have enough pressure on me. Now, there's all this talk about having the *correct* kind of orgasm. Where does all this stuff come from anyway? I'll tell you something. In my day, nobody had an orgasm. And if you did accidentally have one, you were rushed to the hospital.

But now the sexperts tell us that most women are having the *wrong kind* of orgasm. Excuse me? The wrong kind? As opposed to what? I wonder. Yet recent studies have discovered differences between the vaginal, clitoral, and uterine orgasm. Something's left out here. . . . What about the faked orgasm? Does anybody do that one anymore? In my day it was a common practice. But then, that was back in the times when lying in bed meant saying things like "You're the best" or "You're the first."

To make matters worse, the sexual gurus are also saying that one orgasm is *not enough.* If I'm not having multiple orgasms, life is apparently not worth living. Get outta town, gurus. By menopause, I was so prone to bladder infections, yeast infections, and the like, I was worried about having multiple *organisms.* Also, herpes has become so prevalent, they advertise medications like Zamfir on network TV. Gee, I could have sworn that Zamfir is that guy on cable who plays the pan flute. But what do I know?

But wait, there's more. Much, much more. How about all the hoopla over the discovery of a woman's G-spot? No, it's not a guitar chord. It's the anatomical area of a female that is supposed to give her incredibly powerful erotic sensations when stimulated. Sounds good to me. But wait. There's always a catch. This one is that the G-spot is really hard to locate. It poses such a challenge that countless men have made it their career goal to find it. However, few have succeeded, because they refuse to stop and ask for directions.

The thing is, a woman's sexual anatomy is much more complicated than a man's. The G-spot, along with other anatomical structures, is protected by a series of flaps, canals, and muscles. Nature made us this way for our own protection. So it's nearly impossible to find the G-spot without a detailed AAA atlas, a flashlight, and a Sherpa guide. But that doesn't daunt the males species one bit.

You know what I think? This G-spot thing is a bigger hoax than the Loch Ness monster. I don't believe I even have a G-spot, and I told my husband to call off the search. He's not taking charge of any expeditions in my territory.

Men are lucky. They don't have these kinds of problems because everything on them is located right out there in plain sight. That's why a man is so fascinated with his own private parts—they just hang there, like a Chinese lantern.

After all the complaints from men about women's sexual dysfunction, I find it ironic that all the research and medical breakthroughs have only benefited men. That's so typical of our society. I guess maybe we women did it to ourselves, though. They probably figure that if they developed a Viagra pill for women, we'd just fake taking it.

I say let the men have the Viagra. They're welcome to it. Pharmaceutical companies are trying to make it in a spray form, too. I'm not sure whether it will be effective, but it should at least make sneezing a lot more fun. If you ask me, men don't need any more supplemental chemicals or hormone pills. Who knows what could happen? As it is, testosterone causes more than enough indiscriminate behavior in men.

I think I'm better off sticking with natural remedies instead of Viagra-for-women. I'm going to start with soy flour, yam cream, and chasteberries. If they don't work, at least I can always toss a nutritious salad.

After going through menopause, I consider myself a true survivor. Besides menopause, I have survived labor and delivery twice, forty years of periods, PMS, breast cancer, and two Darrens on *Bewitched*. Now, that's what I call a *real* accomplishment.

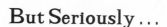

But Seriously...

It's Okay to Slow Down

During menopause, our bodies go through some radical changes. Our estrogen and progesterone levels decrease significantly. So it's perfectly normal for a woman to find that her sex drive is no longer as strong as it was ten years ago. Don't feel as though you are the only one experiencing this, while the rest of the population is out there getting it on every night. Not true. Most loving couples adjust over the years and reach some kind of happy medium.

You don't have to live up to a manufactured image of an oversexed fifty-something vixen. Do you really think Sophia Loren and Carlo Ponti are having wild sex five nights a week? I rest my case.

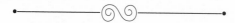

· Quiz ·

Sexual Safari

1. Which phrase do husbands most commonly use when initiating foreplay with love toys?
    a. "Relax, this will be fun."
    b. "I've got a surprise for you."
    c. "Don't peek until I say you can."
    d. "Ladies, start your engines."

2. When making love in a car, which of the following is the most useful marital tool?
    a. a silk blanket
    b. an inflatable pillow
    c. romantic CD's
    d. the jaws of life

3. What do husbands think is the biggest turn-on their wives can wear in the bedroom?
    a. a teddy
    b. a lacy garter belt
    c. nothing
    d. handcuffs

4. Which role might your husband play that would give you twice the action during lovemaking?
    a. Casanova
    b. Rudolph Valentino
    c. Rocky
    d. Dr. Jekyll and Mr. Hyde

5. What role do most husbands want their wives to play?
   a. Marilyn Monroe
   b. the French Maid
   c. Catherine the Great
   d. any nonspeaking one

6. Surreptitious photographs of your husband and some bimbo making love are called . . .
   a. pornography
   b. a turn-on
   c. heartbreaking
   d. exhibit A

7. While making love in broad daylight, middle-aged women request their husbands to put on . . .
   a. a condom
   b. a thong
   c. silk boxers
   d. a blindfold

Quiz Results

The answers to all of the above are d, as in "*do* it!"
   1-3 correct: No cigar.
   4-7 correct: A box of Clinton Cubans.

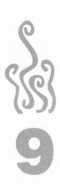

9

MENOPAUSAL MARRIAGES:

Acquisitions and Mergers

Contrary to the opinion of everyone under thirty, there is life after menopause. I didn't dry up from lack of feminine moisture and just blow away. Get real. I only stopped having periods—I haven't stopped living. I don't think Gail Sheehy had a clue when she labeled menopause the "silent passage." All the fifty-somethings I know are as loud as ever. Maybe louder. Hey, come on. I've got a lot of living left to do. I can still get out there and kick up my heels. Sure, I'll probably pull a groin muscle in the process, but what the heck.

Rites of Repetition

I'm just menopausal—not dead. My life did not degenerate into watching soap operas, playing bingo at the VFW, and making attractive bread baskets out of all my leftover tampons. You want to know what my girlfriends and I are doing? We're plenty busy—getting divorced, remarrying, and in some cases getting pregnant again.

This epidemic seems to start in our mid-forties and carry on into our sixties. We keep repeating those rites of passage over and over again. I guess we're going to keep doing it until we get it right. So let this be a warning to all you unattached over-forty males. You guys had better head for the hills. There's an army of women out there, hunting you down, armed with all the tracking ability of the FBI.

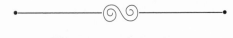

But Seriously ...

Did You Know?

- The number of divorced individuals quadrupled between 1970 and 1996 from 4.3 million to 18.3 million. (National Center for Health Statistics)
- The current divorce rate is .41 percent per capita per year as of 9/6/00. (National Center for Health Statistics)
- 65 percent of new marriages fail. (*Abolition of Marriage* by Maggie Gallagher)
- Of first marriages that end in divorce, many end during the first three to five years. (U.S. Census Bureau)

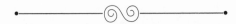

Granted, the second and third time around, the celebrations may take on a slightly different ambience. After all, we can't party the way we did when we were twenty.* But, nonetheless, we're still grabbing all the gusto we legally can. Here's how we menopausals do it:

---

* We can't even remember *being* twenty.

Getting Married . . . Again

Forget about Ellen DeGeneres—I just had a "coming-out" event of my own. Yep. I came out of mothballs to be the world's oldest bridesmaid. My girlfriend Sandy honored me by asking me to be one of four bridesmaids in her beautiful fall wedding. Sandy is in her mid-forties, has a grown son, and has been divorced for many years. This was her second marriage. Her husband-to-be was a widower who also had a son. Anyway, they're a wonderful couple, and I was delighted to be a part of this very happy occasion.

However, even I am inclined to think that the bridesmaid thing needs a cutoff age. Nobody wants to watch an old gal hobbling down the aisle, propped up by two ushers. It's like watching an older flight attendant taking hits of oxygen out of the demo mask.

But Sandy didn't discriminate against the chronologically challenged. She had three bridesmaids in their mid-forties and one in her mid-fifties. That would be me. Guilty as charged. Surprisingly enough, when I told my husband I was going to be a bridesmaid, he was very politically correct about it. I didn't even hear one joke about wearing Depends under my bridesmaid's gown. I found this to be miraculous. Let's be honest here. To a man, menopause is just another opportunity to make insensitive jokes at our expense.

But even though the world can be cruel, we can always count on the women in our lives to show compassion and kindness. This was evidenced by the e-mail my sister shot off to me immediately upon hearing the news: "You—a bridesmaid at your age? Are you joking? Does this mean you'll be in the *Guinness Book of Records*?"

Thanks for sharing. It's great to get those warm fuzzies from family.

The Middle-Aged Bachelorette Party

All of us bridesmaids agreed that Sandy should be given a really boffo bachelorette party. What better way to celebrate her sacred event than by getting totally wasted and acting like morons? Sounds like a plan to me. However, we knew we weren't going to participate in the sort of parties our daughters are having nowadays. We admit it. We're way too old for a wild bachelorette weekend in Vegas, drinking mai tais out of sixty-four-ounce Big Gulps. No getting carried out of the casinos on a stretcher or having our stomachs pumped. No last-minute flings with the Elvis impersonators, either. We no longer have the stamina, the stomachs, or the law school connections it takes to survive one of these events.

We decided on something more age-appropriate, a pool party at my house. We figured we could handle the champagne and canapés. The gals arrived, each carrying a different tray of yummy hors d'oeuvres. We popped them in the oven and headed out to the pool—and the serious business at hand. We uncorked the bubbly and began having lots of girl talk and a lot of laughs. All that girl-bonding stuff was such a high. Like inhaling pure estrogen.

As they say, "Time flies when you're having fun." About two hours later, when we were all pretty much hammered, something unexpected happened. A great-looking guy dressed in a black shirt and pants appeared out of nowhere—a total hunk. He approached us, flashing a badge, claiming he was a fire chief responding to an alarm coming from my house. He had the walkie-talkie, the pager, the ear-wire—the whole thing goin' on.

So naturally what do we forty-something women, all addle-brained from champagne and toxic hormones, think? What else? We all came to the same brilliant conclusion—he was the male stripper hired by one of us bridesmaids to help take this party over the top. We all stood there, fully expecting him to tear off his Velcro uniform and start wildly gyrating his "fire hose" in our faces.

Trust me. There's nothing worse than a bunch of middle-aged women with their inhibitions dangerously lowered by alcohol. So when this man announced for the second time that he was a fire chief, we started smart-mouthing him with stuff like "Oh, sure you are. Let us see your hose." "Really? Why don'tcha put my fire out?" Oh, Lord. You get the picture.

The "fire chief" was not looking even slightly amused. Then, all of a sudden, we heard the wailing siren of a fire truck and tires screeching in my driveway. At this point, our brains were still floating in so much estro-gin, we still didn't comprehend what was really happening. That's when the fire chief led me into my house, which at this point was totally filled with smoke. I couldn't see a foot in front of me.* It was only then that I began to realize I had a teeny-weeny problem.

To make a long story short—you guessed it. The hors d'oeuvres were the culprits. Nuked in the oven for two hours and smoking more than Morton Downey Jr. I had to open every window and door in my house to let it all clear out. But we were troupers. It didn't dampen our resolve. There's always Plan B. So, we grabbed some chips and dip and headed back to the pool. Hey— a minor setback. We still had another two hours and two magnums of champagne to kill.

Second- and Third-Time-Around Weddings

It's a pretty safe bet to assume that a forty- or fifty-year-old bride and groom will each have children and even grandchildren from a previous marriage or marriages. The challenge is to successfully integrate everyone and make a "new" family. Pretty tricky. We're talking about more baggage than American Airlines. These marriages should technically be called mergers. You've got his and her kids, condos, careers, and ex-spouses to negotiate.

That's why I believe men and women in their forties and fifties who are getting remarried should do it in simple civil ceremonies. Let's face it. A second- or third-time-around wedding just doesn't generate the same excitement as a virginal first wedding. Face facts. With these remarriages there is always that "here we go again" feeling in the air.† Why lay on a big, fancy-schmancy wedding for a group of guests who are so skeptical, they're placing bets during the ceremony about how many months your marriage is going to last?

---

* Even without the smoke.
† At Sandy's wedding, instead of the wedding march, they played "The Second Time Around."

No kidding. Even your kids are jaded. Get this. Mark and I were married by a retired rabbi, and invited only our immediate family to a low-key ceremony. It was my third trip down the aisle and his fourth. You heard me right. Between us, we had logged enough miles down the aisle to qualify for frequent-flier points. So you can imagine why our families were less than, shall I say, enthusiastic. But the crowning blow was delivered by Mark's five-year-old daughter. As we were leaving the temple, she waved good-bye to the rabbi and said, "See you the next time my daddy gets married." It took approximately three hours for everyone to stop laughing.

Is it any wonder I am telling you to keep it low-key? Here's my list of reasons why an older couple getting married for the second, third, or fourth time should not have a big wedding:

- Your new husband is so broke from paying alimony and child support to his ex, all you can afford is a cold buffet at Denny's.
- His hostile ex-wife will continually threaten to phone in a bomb threat on your wedding day.
- The kids from both marriages have officially declared war on each other.
- All your friends expect it to fail, so they send chintzy gifts, enclosing the sales slips for quick returns.
- Most guests will send "regrets" with excuses ranging from prostate surgery to alien abductions.
- The only person who will agree to perform the ceremony is a New Age guru wearing a white robe, and crystals around his neck.

Believe me, there's a lot of truth to this. At my age, I've been to every conceivable type of middle-aged wedding. I went to one where the forty-five-year-old bride was six months pregnant and wore a full-length white wedding gown. Mercy. Priscilla of Boston was probably turning over in her grave.

The best one, though, was a second-time-around wedding on a ship that was presided over by the English captain. When the bride said, "I do," he replied, "Is that your *final* answer?" Big yuks all around.

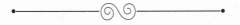

But Seriously ...

Second Helpings

Even though the statistics on the success of second and higher marriages are pretty sobering, I remain the eternal optimist. From my experience, we're a lot more grounded and committed to making the marriage work at midlife than when we were younger. We're also sorely aware of what was lacking in our previous marriage or marriages and are very appreciative of having it now.

I have found that when these later-in-life marriages hit some bumps, the couples are more willing to go to counseling. Maybe it's just because we have more disposable income at this age, or more time, or maybe it's because we know this marriage is our "last chance." But whatever the reason, it seems to hold true for the couples I know.

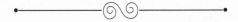

· Quiz ·

Perilous Passages

1. When both partners in a couple have been married twice before, who is the most appropriate person to conduct their ceremony?
   a. a justice of the peace
   b. a minister
   c. a captain of a ship
   d. an Elvis impersonator

2. When marrying for the third time, what should you budget for as your biggest expense?
   a. a new home
   b. the wedding reception
   c. the honeymoon
   d. alimony

3. The night before the wedding, many men surprise their brides-to-be with a . . .
   a. trip to Bali
   b. two-carat-diamond necklace
   c. brand-new SUV
   d. prenup

4. When the bachelorette party is over, it's customary for the bride to leave . . .
   a. first
   b. in a limo
   c. before midnight
   d. in an ambulance

5. Every woman attending the bachelorette party would pay any amount of money to have which magnum on her lips?
   a. Dom Perignon
   b. Veuve Cliquot
   c. Taittinger
   d. P.I.

6. You're probably partying too hard when your next event requires . . .
   a. financing
   b. a caterer
   c. a bartender
   d. an intervention

7. For a menopausal woman, eating too much, drinking too much, and compulsive shopping are signs that she's having . . .
   a. a mental breakdown
   b. fluctuating hormones
   c. depression
   d. a perfect day

Quiz Results
The answers to all of the above are d, as in "Dry out."
   1–3 correct: Keep taking those baby steps.
   4–7 correct: You'll need the 12 steps.

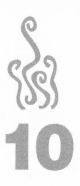

10

TEST-TUBE PREGNANCY:

"Honey, I Defrosted the Kids!"

Ten . . . nine . . . eight . . . seven . . . six . . . The countdown is on. Uh-oh, Houston, we've got a problem. Time is running out. According to my latest follicle-stimulating-hormone test, I've got three months, six days, and seven minutes left before I'm officially out of the egg business.

It Ain't Over till It's Over

As they say, "All good things must come to an end." They also say, "The best is yet to come." Wow. How profound that is. But who the heck are "they"? I have no idea. Never did. However, I do know this. It's time for me to take stock of my life so far. I should count my blessings for all the wonderful things I have:

1. Healthy, well-adjusted kids who did well in college.
2. A beautiful home with the mortgage paid off.
3. A loving husband who is happy with his family and his job.

4. More time to pursue my life-long interests.

5. The opportunity to travel and see the world.

Wrap your mind around this: For me menopause was a totally liberating experience. From where I stand, I'd say the past, present, and future look pretty darned rosy. I've thrown away all my Midol and diuretics. I've finally gotten rid of the two biggest headaches of my life:

1. Periods

2. Birth control

That's right. Just think about it. You are never going to suffer through another period *for the rest of your lives*! Let that sink in for a moment. Do you get it, or do I have to act it out with a sock puppet? Pretty heavy stuff. More profound than the Elton John–Eminem duet. But just in case you have even a teeny-weeny feeling of regret, think back to those days when your cramps were so bad, you had to drag a Midol IV around.

Flood Insurance

I have finally come to understand what that "oh, so fresh feeling" is. But something I will never understand is this: How come scientific technology put a man on the moon and cracked the code of DNA, but never invented a tampon that *didn't leak*? Beats me. It's not exactly rocket science. And because of scientists' incompetence, I was forced to wear a supersized tampon with a backup pad the size of a Sealy Posturepedic mattress. Give me a break. I carried around more packing than a UPS parcel.

On my heavy days, I had to wear *two* super tampons at the same time. Even so, after a few hours they developed stress fractures. What a miserable feeling that was! Forget PMS. No wonder I was in such a bad mood for a week. I couldn't walk three feet without taking a Darvon. It was hard enough getting two of them in, but getting them out was murder. It required the Heimlich maneuver. Is it any wonder I say "Good riddance!"

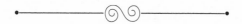

Remember the Old-Fashioned Sanitary Belt?

You needed a degree from MIT just to figure out how to wear it.

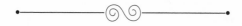

As I see it, there is only one downside to not having a period, and that is not having a convenient excuse to beg off from sex when we aren't in the mood. It was the one excuse that worked 100 percent of the time. Why? Because of the universal irony of men's behavior. On one hand, they can't get enough blood and guts in the movies. When Mel Gibson got disemboweled in *Braveheart,* they were in heaven. When Joe Pesci bludgeoned five guys to death in *Casino,* they watched in utter fascination. And the pièce de résistance was *Hannibal* where Anthony Hopkins served up Ray Liotta's brain* with some fava beans and a bottle of good chianti.

But when it comes to a close encounter with a little menstrual flow, the he-men get all weak in the knees and back off like you have leprosy.

I've Got Rhythm

Even better than not having your period is not having to worry about birth control anymore. It seems like the responsibility for birth control has always been left up to women. It still is, for that matter. Even in this day and age, most of the birth control available still has a lot of problems. Women bear all the discomfort and the risk in exchange for giving men most of the pleasure. If you ask me, that's a worse deal than Linda Tripp's severance package.

---

* Al dente.

The things we've put up with:
    The IUD
    The diaphragm
    The female condom
    Contraceptive foam
    Spermicidal gel
    The cervical sponge
    The pill
    Tubal ligation

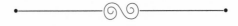

But Seriously ...

Cancer and Contraception

If you have been diagnosed with breast cancer and have not yet reached menopause, there are a lot of factors to be considered when you choose birth control. If the tumor is estrogen-receptive (grows in the presence of estrogen), you will not be able to take birth control pills because they contain estrogen.

Chemotherapy can put an end to normal ovarian function, resulting in an earlier onset of menopause, which eliminates the need for contraception. You will need to discuss these issues with your oncologist and gynecologist. They will help you arrive at a decision that best suits your circumstances.

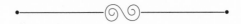

There is one birth control method that is perfect for us women. It is not a medication that endangers our health or makes us bloated. It is not any type of female surgery. It isn't messy or painful—and it's 100 percent effective. It's the answer to a woman's prayers. Sounds too good to be true, eh? What is it? A *vasectomy*.

Surprise, surprise! All you have to do is figure out how to talk your husband into it. What are the odds of doing that? Probably the same as him voting for the acquittal of Lorena Bobbitt. But it's worth the effort. Keep after him until he agrees. You can always issue this ultimatum: "No splice—no dice!"

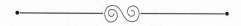

But Seriously...

His or Hers?

My husband decided to have a vasectomy when we got married, because he was in his late forties and already had four daughters. He had it done in a urologist's office under a local anesthetic. The recuperation period was twenty-four hours, and he went back to work the next day. He says it was "a piece of cake."

We were in agreement that this was the best solution for us. We both had grown kids, and were absolutely certain we weren't going to have any more. For me, it was not only a welcome solution but also a practical one. A tubal ligation, in which a woman is rendered infertile by "tying off" the fallopian tubes, is also an outpatient procedure, but it involves slightly more risk and recovery time.

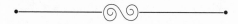

What Was I Thinking?

If you can't get your husband to snip and clip, you may be in trouble, because wild hormonal fluctuations also deprive women's brains of vital oxygen. As a result, too many fall victim to a certain kind of "rational" thinking that goes something like this:

"Let's see. I'm a happy, healthy forty-six-year-old woman. I've got a great life and lots of free time. What else could I possibly want? Of course, that's it! Another baby."

Is this scary or what? We're listening to a classic case of temporary insanity caused by toxic hormone levels. How else could a woman come up with this decision? She really thinks having another baby at that age will bring her total fulfillment? Well, think again. Before you let your hormones lead you down that path of no return, ask yourself these questions:

Do you want to stay awake every night for the next year breastfeeding an infant? Are you nuts? Think about it. Our menopausal breasts are saggy enough as it is. And now, you're going to engorge them with six quarts of milk? Are you kidding? By the time you deliver, you'll be wearing a 46-long nursing bra.

Do you really want to spend the next three years changing diapers? Remember this factoid: Every hour, infants poop their own body weight into their diapers. Not to mention the aroma wafting through your house from a Diaper Genie sitting in every room. And this after being nauseated through the whole nine months of pregnancy?

Also, don't forget that osteoporosis is a major problem in midlife. You'd better pray that your menopausal hip doesn't snap like a twig from carrying your baby around on it all day long. According to my calculations, I'm not due for a hip replacement for another twenty years, or 7,000 miles.

And what about your beautiful home? You've spent the last fifteen years decorating it to perfection. Do you really want to transform it from *House Beautiful* to a Toys "R" Us junkyard? It will happen before you can say *Sesame Street*. From now on you won't have a piece of furniture or a square inch of carpet that isn't stained with strained peas, squash, carrots, or worse.

Are you ready to cope with a baby screaming at the top of his or her lungs in public places? Especially on an airplane, when everybody is trying to sleep and your baby is wailing for six hours, nonstop? Just look around at the expressions on your fellow passengers' faces. Feel the love.

Forget about your IRA, savings account, and the money market. They're toast. Nowadays, schools are so expensive, you'll have to take out a second mortgage just to finance grades K through 6 in private school. And if the school has a name with "country day" in it, make it another fifty grand.

Unless you still have your head buried in your yam cream, I think you can see where this saga is going. Now, far be it from me to rain on your parade. I don't mean to sound completely negative and preachy. So if you're one of those middle-aged women who are seriously entertaining thoughts about having another baby—I'll say this as gently and supportively as I can: ARE YOU OUT OF YOUR FREAKIN' MIND? GET OVER IT!

There, I feel better. You will, too, after you have a couple of margaritas to clear your head. Better yet, have the whole pitcher. Just know that pregnancy in your forties or early fifties is no walk in the park. It's more like navigating a minefield. But if you still think the whole thing is going to be fun and games, keep reading. Here are some options for menopausal women who might encounter difficulties conceiving:

Fun at the Fertility Clinic

This is the place for women who are down to their last couple of eggs. That, or their husbands have sperm counts lower than the IQ's of World Wrestling Federation fans. These clinics have doctors who specialize in fertility problems, and they can perform miracles even in the toughest cases.

But be forewarned. You're about to embark on a roller-coaster ride more intense than the Apollo Chariot at Busch Gardens. Here's what happened to my girlfriend Lucy.

The doctors started by requesting a sperm sample from her husband, to make sure his sperm count was adequate. In the old days, this would have been like taking candy from a baby. But those days are over. At his age, sperm is a rare commodity. It's not like when you were in college and there was so much of it around, you were tripping over it. When the nurse sends him into a clinically sterile room with a plastic cup, a copy of *Playboy,* and a video, Lucy knows what to expect. He might as well take *Mission Impossible* in there with him.

Despite the challenge to Lucy's husband, however, most of the medical procedures were done on her. She was the main event. Basically, the doctors were trying to jump-start two ovaries that were nearing their expiration date. They were pumping her with all kinds of hormones, and didn't quit until she was producing more eggs than Frank Purdue's chicken farms.

Of course, when she was taking hormones, there was the little matter of side effects. Did I hear anybody mention the word "bloating"? Trust me. She didn't hear it from her doctors. All they said was that she might experience some "slight swelling." Uh-huh . . . She was retaining more water than the Hoover Dam. Talk about swollen ankles. She actually bought stock in a queen-panty-hose company.*

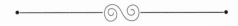

But Seriously . . .

"Be Prepared"—a Great Motto

Educate yourself about infertility before embarking upon treatment. I know from many of my girlfriends' experiences that fertility treatments can be a long and difficult road. It can put a big strain on a woman emotionally and physically, and often on the marriage, too.

Don't get me wrong. I am all for doing whatever it takes to have a baby. What I am saying is that you need to prepare yourself and be completely knowledgeable about what you are going to be going through. The more understanding you have about the process, the better you'll be able to cope with the difficulties as they arise.

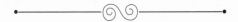

* From a drag queen.

Uh-Oh, I'm Ovulating

Once the hormones started working, Lucy's next task was to figure out exactly when she would be ovulating. There is only a small window of time, usually less than twenty-four hours, when the egg can be fertilized. To pinpoint when ovulation would take place, she was given a kit to test her cervical mucus. Yep, you heard me right. And no, don't ask me anything else about it. I don't even want to think about what she was supposed to do with it.

An easier method was to take her temperature at regular intervals, because it spikes slightly during ovulation. It was such a trip seeing her in the fertility clinic. She and a bunch of other menopausal women had thermometers clamped in their mouths and ovulation charts pinned to their chests. As if this wasn't bad enough, some even had gray hair and grandchildren. I just don't think I could handle being part of a fertility group that looks like the road company from *Cocoon*.

The big moment occurred when her doctor suspected she was ovulating. All hell broke loose. The egg has landed. "One small step for man. . . ." Now she was down to the wire. The race was on to get that little sucker fertilized. And naturally, the one time you need a man, he's never around. But even if he was in Nepal meditating with Richard Gere,* guaranteed he'd jump on the nearest yak and get his fanny home—stat.

Then they had to do it—do it—do it—night and day, in hopes that one of those little guys would make it to the finish line and fertilize her egg. Did you know that it takes millions of sperm to fertilize one egg? That's because they won't stop and ask for directions.

Normally sex is an enjoyable thing. But for Lucy, it was more like an endurance test. Survival of the fittest, baybee. If you ask me, having sex three or four times in a day isn't natural. I don't know about you, but at my age, I'm not into sexual gymnastics. I have a problem just getting out of bed in the morning. And I

* In an Armani sarong.

haven't even mentioned the added risks like overexposure and terminal abrasions. *Oy vey.* Pass the Advil and K-Y jelly.

Taking the Shortcut

There are many couples of all ages who are unable to go the traditional route of having a baby. Fortunately, now there are a variety of technical detours that will take them to the same destination.

In Vitro Fertilization

This is a technique in which a woman's eggs are harvested* from her own ovaries, fertilized in a petri dish with her husband's or a donor's sperm, and implanted in her uterus. Her body has been primed with hormones that allow her uterus to support the embryo to full term.

Often, several fertilized eggs are transferred at the same time. This raises the odds of at least one of the embryos making it to full term. In many cases, more than one of the fertilized eggs survives, resulting in a multiple birth.†

If a woman's uterus is not able to support the pregnancy, she may decide to have the embryo implanted into the uterus of a cooperative, loving surrogate.‡

Yes, it's a new reproductive world out there. A single woman can bear her own child by being inseminated with sperm from a donor of her choosing. There is even the option of surfing the Net for donor sperm or eggs.§ They offer detailed genetic histories of the donors available for study.

Marriage is no longer a prerequisite for childbirth. All it takes is a donor and a freezer. The phrase "out of wedlock" has become obsolete. It has been replaced by the more appropriate "out of Ziploc."

* Using machinery manufactured by John Deere.
† Just call it a litter.
‡ After she signs the 500-page legal contract drawn up by her six lawyers.
§ www.eggsrus.com

I admit I have problems with this technique. It's just so "out there." It's too much like a *Star Wars* episode for me. Just think about it. If you are impregnated with somebody else's egg and sperm, you're giving birth to someone you're not related to. Is that weird or what?

Wow! Isn't this miraculous technology? There are so many choices about conception available to a woman. She no longer has to put all her eggs in one basket.

Frozen Follies

There are institutions that keep eggs and sperm frozen indefinitely. Sometimes, younger couples opt to have their eggs and sperm frozen for future use. A man might decide to have his sperm frozen before a vasectomy, in case he changes his mind about having more children at a later date. Or some twenty-year-old changes it for him.

Some women even have an egg fertilized, then frozen. This way, their offspring are available when they're ready. No more waiting. No muss, no fuss. Childbirth becomes a simple matter. In a modern household, you may well hear someone exclaim, "Honey, I defrosted the kids."

Menopausal mamas are popping up all over the place. Is this a good thing or a bad thing? Hey—far be it from me to pass judgment. You won't hear any snide or discouraging comments from me. What's that? I said *what* in *which* chapter? Well, excuuuuuse me. I'm going through menopause, so I don't remember saying any of it!

To any woman contemplating motherhood during midlife, I say good luck and Godspeed. Please let me know if there is anything I can do for you. As a women's advocate and staunch female supporter, I'll be happy to support you in any decision you make.

Feel free to ask me any favor. There's nothing I wouldn't do to help out another woman. Ummm—wait a minute. You mentioned baby-sitting? Sorry—I must have had another one of my "menopausal moments."

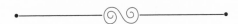

But Seriously ...

Conception After Cancer

We are lucky to be living in an age when fertility technology is so advanced that we have options our mothers never dreamed of. Women who have experienced early-onset menopause and even those who have had ovarian cancer can still have children through the miracles of modern technology.

There are also increasing numbers of breast cancer patients who will go on to have babies, whereas years ago this was highly discouraged. Better treatment and knowledge of the disease have made this option available. The gorgeous and talented Ann Jillian, who had a double mastectomy, is just one example of that success.

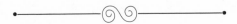

The Advanced Baby Shower

I never thought that when I reached the age I am now, I'd be getting invited to baby showers every other week. And not all of them are for my friends' daughters. Thanks to the miracles of modern technology, most of them are for my own girlfriends, many of whom are in their second or third marriages.

Other times, these preganancies are midlife accidents. Talk about being depressed. You won't find any of these women jumping for joy. It's more like they're jumping off the second-floor balcony. No wonder they say most accidents happen at home. Unfortunately, 99 percent of them are in the bedroom.

It's also not uncommon for women going through the change of life to overmedicate themselves. Many of them confuse their birth control pills with their Valium. The bad news is that one day, they find themselves menopausal and pregnant. But the good news is, they don't give a damn.

So, let's take a minute to review our menopause lesson. Repeat after me: "Menopause is the most fulfilling time of my life." Just think—now you can enjoy a life of complete freedom:

No kids
No period
More sex
Well, two out of three ain't bad.

· Quiz ·

Midlife Mistakes

1. The first time you resume sex after delivering a midlife baby, what should you keep by your bedside?
   a. a box of condoms
   b. a bottle of Advil
   c. a tube of Astroglide
   d. an anesthesiologist

2. Which of the following locations has the most plentiful donor sperm?
   a. a sperm bank
   b. an Internet auction
   c. a fertility clinic
   d. David Crosby's house

3. Who will pay the astronomical cost incurred by a sixty-three-year-old woman giving birth?
   a. Medicare
   b. Blue Cross/Blue Shield
   c. the state
   d. the *National Enquirer*

4. Most new seventy-five-year-old fathers are willing to take the 3 A.M. feeding shift because they . . .
   a. are so grateful for the baby
   b. need less sleep at their age
   c. want to experience the bonding
   d. get up to pee every hour anyway

5. When a single, middle-aged woman desperately wants to find a husband and have a baby, which team of specialists should she consult first?
   a. fertility specialists
   b. neonatal pediatricians
   c. high-risk-pregnancy obstetricians
   d. cosmetic surgeons

6. When you are thinking about pregnancy later in life, which body part should you have frozen first?
   a. your eggs
   b. your husband's sperm
   c. your blood platelets
   d. your brain

7. Three days after giving birth, which medical procedure is requested by 99 percent of middle-aged mothers?
   a. episiotomy repair
   b. hemorrhoidectomy
   c. D and C
   d. vasectomy

Quiz Results

The answers to all of the above are d, as in "Demerol."

1–3 correct: Thirty years' hard labor.

4–7 correct: Stay of execution.

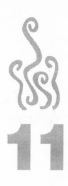

11

LIFE AFTER MENOPAUSE:

The Angina Monologues

I am often asked, "What is the hardest time of a woman's life?" My answer: "Birth to death." It's true. We barely have time to recover from pregnancies and giving birth when we're jolted into menopause and parboiled with hot flashes. Not to mention the forty years we've spent doubled over with cramps from our "friend." Some friend. Like Linda Tripp.

And men. My husband has no sympathy for my female troubles, because he's never had to go through anything like them. The only thing he had to suffer through that was even remotely close was a prostate exam. And even then, he requested a general anesthetic. Men have no clue as to the kind of maintenance a woman's body requires. While we spend half of our lives cleansing, medicating, and irrigating our body parts, all men do is stand around scratching theirs.

Most people believe that one of a woman's toughest physical challenges is giving birth. Not true. It's afterward, when you try to resume your sex life. In a word—agony. It requires the same physical stamina as a three-hour performance of Riverdance.* We know that it's going to hurt like hell, so we keep putting it off—like until we die from natural causes.

But sooner or later, we have to face the music.† So I say, make it easy on yourselves. Take a few painkillers. It will certainly help get you through this ordeal. And don't worry about reaching that sexual peak. The real challenge is to stay conscious for the first five minutes.

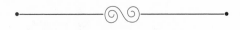

But Seriously...

Looking Ahead

Menopausal women don't look anything like they did in our mothers' day. We have the advantage of being able to prevent many of the problems associated with old age, from heart disease to osteoporosis. We are acutely aware of the benefits regular exercise gives our inner and outer bodies. Both men and women aren't dying of cancer, diabetes, and stroke as they did just twenty or thirty years ago.

I love not being encumbered with a period every month. It leaves me free to exercise and travel with no interruption. Thanks to routine medical testing, advanced medical techniques, a good diet, and regular exercise, I expect to live well into my nineties. I am not kidding when I say that now, after menopause and breast cancer, I am healthier than I have ever been before.

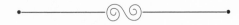

* Executed in the nude.
† And the ceiling.

The Postmenopausal Lifestyle

But I digress. Let's look ahead to life after menopause. And yes, there is a life. We may not be out there cycling with Lance Armstrong or playing doubles with Venus Williams, but we've still got a lot of life left in us. We just have to change our activities a little, to accommodate muscles with less tone than Bob Dylan. But we don't have to become spectators. Here are some of the kinds of activities we postmenopausals can still participate in:

Scrabble. Don't count me out. I may not be able to run the four-minute mile, but I've still got a fabulous memory. Now what was it I wanted to tell you about? Oh, yeah, Scrabble. Postmenopausals can get so expert that many reach tournament level. How so? Well, at my age, I have quadrupled my vocabulary. I can wipe out the competition with my knowledge of words like "osteoporosis," "pneumothorax," "thrombosis," "fibromyalgia," and "ischemia." Ooooh—remembering all those words just gave me a headache. Does anybody have an ibuprofen?

Mah-jongg. The only prerequisite for this game is nine-inch acrylic fingernails. Also, they must be filed to the point where they're registered as lethal weapons. These nails will provide that extra competitive edge, as they fly across the tiles at warp speed.

To successfully play in a mah-jongg game, the only thing that has to be sharper than your nails is your tongue. This is because 99 percent of the game consists of vicious gossip. Women tend to spill their guts in the hairdresser's chair and at the mah-jongg table. So, when I'm playing this game, I'm always prepared to dish! I've been a party to stories of dirty divorce sagas and family infidelities, and I've learned about more illegitimate children than Jesse Jackson's. It's a regular shtup-fest.

There's just one word of caution. If the discussion gets too raunchy for you, do not put your fingers in your ears.

Bowling. After menopause, the bowling leagues will hunt you down with the skill of Army recruiters. And once you let them into your house, you're dead meat. They use more subversive tactics than the Branch Davidians.

Bowling leagues operate from a cult mentality. In no time after joining, I was proudly wearing my league jacket everywhere. Naturally, it's black silk with the league name, "Premarin Panthers," embroidered across the back. I also had to buy my own personalized leather bag to carry my custom-made ball. Also, no self-respecting leaguer would be caught dead in rental shoes. Nobody wants to wear those grungy things that have been rubbing against someone else's corn plasters for the last ten years.

The big plus about bowling is that I don't have to be in prime physical shape to be good at it. With the potent combination of cortisone and Coors coursing through my veins, I'm able to bowl strikes off my big toe.

Bingo. This game is quite popular with older people, because it doesn't require an athletic body. Basically, all it takes is one flexible digit and a state of consciousness. Retired women flock to bingo parlors seven days a week. And they become so skillful, they're able to handle ten cards at once.

When I sit in on one of these games, I never take those blue-haired ladies for granted. They go for the jugular. They win all the jackpots before the younger players have time to locate G-45 on one card. What a confidence builder. At least in their old age, they've finally been able to locate their G-spots.

Coupon clipping. This qualifies as an activity, because it takes at least two muscle groups to cut coupons out of the newspaper. After the kids left home, we didn't feel much like cooking anymore. Eating out became a way of life. Therefore, much of my free time is spent going through magazines and *Penny Savers*, locating coupons for early-bird specials and two-fers.

That's why I have become a staunch supporter of that great American institution, the salad bar. It offers everything I'm looking for: good prices, low-calorie selections, and that all-important sneeze-guard. About the only thing they're short on is nutrition. But, hey, you can't have everything.

For $5.95 I get to heap a mountain of warm lettuce on a chilled plate. Then I get to choose from a vast array of nutritionally inert toppings like rubberized bacon bits and croutons harder than Dick Cheney's arteries.

A special crowd pleaser is the side dish of pickled beets containing enough red dye number 3 to turn my urine pink for a week. But that's okay with me. I'm not big on those organic health foods. I figure at my age, I need all the preservatives I can get.

Long-Term Maintenance Contracts

Now, if you're thinking that life after menopause is merely a series of early-bird specials, you're wrong. I also spend a good deal of my time trying to maintain good health. In fact, I keep my doctors on speed dial. Used parts require a lot of maintenance. Nowadays my priorities have shifted. I need a smaller house and a bigger medicine cabinet.

Here's the round-robin of doctors I see during an average month:

The G.P. No matter how many specialists I have, I still love our old family doc the best. Yes, he probably should have hung up his stethoscope in the late 1950s.* But he makes me feel safe and secure—like being with my grandpa again. So no matter how old and doddering he gets, I'm sticking to him like Polygrip.

The dermatologist. Unfortunately, now I'm paying the price for all the years I spent baking in the sun. Remember those days when we slathered on the baby oil and iodine, then sat in the direct sunlight with a reflecting shield propped under our chins? Does the phrase "human barbecue" mean anything to you? Man, oh, man. After a couple of hours of sunbathing like this, I could only be identified by my dental records.

In those days everybody's goal was to get a George Hamilton tan. But believe me, I never looked as pretty as he did. On the contrary. And look at those old gals in Florida, who have spent a lifetime baking in the sun. At this point, they're so leathery, they've been declared an endangered species.

---

* Now it doubles as his hearing aid.

A dermatologist can easily treat most sun-damaged areas with a can of frozen nitrogen. He or she sprays it on age spots, keratoses, and other growths. After a few days, these areas scab over and fall off. But even though the treatment isn't that bad, I still blame George Hamilton for setting such a bad example. I'd like to spray that nitrogen down his pants and wait for the same results.

The cardiologist. When I got past fifty, I became positively obsessed with the old ticker. So now I'm adding a cardiologist and a cardiac surgeon to my ever-growing database of medical maintenance personnel. These men may literally hold my life in their hands one day. If that isn't scary enough, the worst part is, they both look like my twenty-five-year-old son.

But at some point, they will probably extend my life with innovative procedures like an angiogram, an angioplasty, an endarterectomy, and bypass surgery. These procedures clear out clogged arteries and reduce the chance of future heart attacks. A cardiac surgeon has the skill to replace damaged heart valves, or graft new vessels onto the heart itself. Impressive. These procedures can not only extend my life but also improve the quality of my life.

However, you ain't heard nothin' yet. Recently, they have perfected a totally artificial heart for implantation in humans. It's going to virtually eliminate the need for donors. I'm not sure what the global implications will be, but I do know what this means for the women in L.A.: There will be thousands of them walking around who don't have a single original body part left!

Think of it. With medical advances like these, I might be living to 150 or longer. Even without these medical miracles, people nowadays are living much longer. Better nutrition, state-of-the-art health care, and renewed interest in exercise have already increased our life spans. There are thousands of men and women living past 100 right now.

Actually, I knew one. He was my parents' neighbor in Florida. He died at 102! I'm not sure what was the official cause of death, though. I think he overslept and they buried him.

I'm learning more and more about the important role genetics plays in longevity. Thank your lucky stars if you have parents and grandparents who have lived a long, healthy life. Chances are that with a little luck and good medical care, you can also live to a ripe old age. I know when my time comes, though, I want to go peacefully in my sleep the way my grandfather did—not like his screaming passengers.

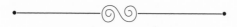

But Seriously . . .

Taking Charge

After I emerged from menopause and my bout with cancer, one thing became crystal clear. I am totally responsible for keeping myself healthy. My doctors are wonderful, but their job is just to monitor my health with their tests. The real job is up to me. I accomplish this through regular exercise, a diet of organic foods, and meditation to relieve stress.

In addition, I have regular checkups. They can catch any condition early, when it is easiest to treat. That's why it's so important to have a mammogram and a Pap smear and see your internist at least once a year.

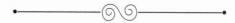

The Pause That Refreshes

I think we need to celebrate menopause. What do you say? Let's do it. I kind of like being part of a generation whose primary focus is feminine moisture replacement. Here are some ideas for making menopause a blast:

Age-Appropriate Gifts
Any battery-operated marital aid
Giant-sized tube of Astroglide
Case of Depends
Economy-size Metamucil
Six months of anger-management classes
Lifetime supply of Flexall
Gift certificate for a colonoscopy

Age-Appropriate Activities
Creating a bonfire of Tampax
Timing our hot flashes
Group instruction in Kegel exercise technique
Group crying jag
Sparring match between two menopausal women

Age-Appropriate Menu
Herbal tea with soy milk
Soybean salad with flaxseed-oil dressing
Eggless tofu salad
Anything loaded with bran
Prune juice smoothie

If anyone ever deserved a party, it's a menopausal woman. But please, let me celebrate in my own way. I don't want to hear any criticism from you twenty- and thirty-somethings. It's my party and I'll cry if I want to. You would cry too if it happened to you.

• Quiz •

Golden Girls

1. The medical profession has been in serious trouble since . . .
   a. HMO's appeared
   b. insurance companies got tough
   c. hospital costs skyrocketed
   d. George Clooney left

2. What is the one thing menopausal women fear most?
   a. being widowed
   b. being put in an old-age home
   c. a terminal disease
   d. their proctologist

3. Which one of the following do most men over sixty try to emulate?
   a. Billy Graham
   b. John Glenn
   c. Dr. Christian Barnard
   d. Strom Thurmond

4. How does your body tell you that you've had enough sun?
   a. Your mouth gets dry.
   b. You develop a headache.
   c. You experience blurred vision.
   d. Your belly button pops up.

5. If you're retired, your kids will feel better when you're living in a safe place like a . . .
   a. gated community
   b. high-rise apartment building
   c. house with an alarm system
   d. maximum-security rest home

6. The most serious malady among the elderly population in Florida is . . .
   a. heart attack
   b. stroke
   c. diabetes
   d. dangling chads

7. The newest technological feature built into all of the latest artificial hearts is . . .
   a. titanium valves
   b. Gore-Tex vessels
   c. state-of-the-art wiring
   d. E-mail

Quiz Results

The answers to all of the above are d, as in "Depends."

    1–3 correct: Not really incompetent.

    4–7 correct: Most likely incontinent.

12

BUT SERIOUSLY . . .

My Personal Journey with Cancer

I'm going to switch gears and get serious. For a long time now, I have debated whether I should even relate this story. I'm a humor writer, and everybody expects me to be funny all the time. But the truth is that life isn't always a barrel of laughs. Bad things happen to funny people, too. Although breast and ovarian cancer aren't necessarily related to menopause, many women are diagnosed during that time in their lives. So I decided that my experience was especially relevant to this book, because it happened to me during menopause. My hope is that you will gain knowledge and strength from my personal story. After all, we're all in this together.

It was a gorgeous, sunny August afternoon in 1997. My girl-friend Linda Wexler and I were having lunch to celebrate our budding careers. Linda had just self-published the first in a series of books about places to go for tea. She was establishing herself as the "tea lady" on the West Coast and building a whole new career around it. Her book sales were going great guns.

I had recently signed with a female literary agent in New

York who was optimistic about selling my new manuscript to a major publisher. My *Hormones from Hell* had been translated into seven languages, and it was going to be released in a hard-cover edition in Germany. I was going to Frankfurt in October, to sign at the International Book Expo.

Linda and I were so excited about our futures. Our lives were, as they say, about as good as it gets. All the hard work was finally starting to pay off. Our dreams were starting to come true. How could we know that in a few short weeks, we'd both be diagnosed with cancer, shattering all our dreams? Even worse—one of us wasn't going to make it.

It was September when Linda called with the horrifying news. She had been experiencing some vague abdominal pains for a while, but lately they had become really severe. After a week of medical tests, a CAT scan revealed the worst. She had a ten-centimeter tumor on her ovary. The doctors were 99 percent sure that it was malignant. And because of its size, they were not optimistic about her prognosis. As I listened to her talking, it was almost as though I was going into another reality. I was totally stunned. Speechless. We both started crying. I tried to reassure her, but my words sounded hollow. There are times when reality is so ugly and frightening, you are rendered totally helpless.

Just before I left for Frankfurt, Linda had her surgery. The news was not good. The tumor was an aggressive mixed mesothelioma, which is a particularly tough one to kill off. Within a week of the surgery, she began an aggressive course of chemotherapy. Time was of the essence. We talked on the phone every day, and I tried to be her cheerleader in those dark, dark days.

Meanwhile, I hadn't been feeling so great myself. There were a lot of things going on in my body that I hadn't experienced before. For the past few months I had been having mega-menopausal night sweats that would have me waking up totally soaked. Before this, they had been milder and less drenching. I found that my immune system was breaking down. I traveled a lot to promote my books, and it seemed as though every time I went on a trip I'd come down with a bad head cold or the flu. I was also having odd problems with my feet. I was experiencing a lot of pain in one of my heels, and I couldn't seem to get rid of it. I went through three pairs of new gym shoes and many heel cushions, but nothing worked.

I was sick as a dog when my husband and I came back from Frankfurt and London. A massive cold had hit me halfway through our trip. I vowed that when I got home, I would cut down on my travels and start taking better care of myself.

Because I have had fibrocystic breast disease since my early thirties, I've always been diligent about going for checkups. Fibrocystic breast disease is basically a benign condition in which the breast tissue periodically forms fluid-filled cysts. The condition is a result of fluctuating hormone levels—specifically, estrogen is the culprit. I noticed that on the months I had really heavy periods, I was more likely to form a cyst. However, caffeine from coffee, chocolate, or other foods can also promote flare-ups.

I saw a breast surgeon, Dr. Mitchell Karlan, twice a year, who aspirated these cysts fairly regularly. I also saw my gynecologist twice a year. I was going through menopause and was taking low-dosage birth control pills to help alleviate its symptoms. I had a mammogram once a year, like clockwork. In fact, I had had one five months before my November appointment with my gynecologist, Dr. Sharon Winer.

During my exam, Dr. Winer felt a lumpy area in my right breast. This wasn't all that unusual for me. So, although I wasn't happy, I wasn't hysterical either. However, I immediately went to Dr. Karlan. He aspirated it, but only a tiny amount of fluid came out. Not the usual two cubic centimeters. This was a little unsettling, but still, I left his office relieved that I'd had it taken care of.

The next morning when I took the bandage off to shower, I instinctively put my hand on my right breast. I expected it to feel nice and flat where the cyst had been. Instead, I felt a lump still there. In the fifteen years that I had been getting these cysts aspirated, this had never happened before. I broke out in a cold sweat.

I looked at my breast in the mirror, and noticed something that really shook me. The skin over the lump was the tiniest bit "striated" looking. I knew that one of the signs of breast cancer is dimpling of the skin or a stippled effect, like the skin of an orange. Doctors even have a name for this, *peau d'orange*. Mine wasn't exactly either of these, but there was a slight difference in the skin texture from that of my other breast.

I went back to Dr. Karlan. The signs looked good. I had no history of breast cancer in my family, and the lump was small and soft to the touch. The fluid from the cyst showed no malignant cells. But just to be sure, he wanted to do a biopsy. The next morning he did the procedure under a local anesthetic. We were both in a pretty good mood, because basically neither of us believed the lump was cancerous. We even told each other some jokes as he was getting started. I guess I felt that, somehow, if I could laugh through the whole thing, nothing bad would happen to me.

But as time passed he became silent. When he finally spoke, it was to say he was just about finished. But he didn't add, "It's nothing," or "It looks good," or "Don't worry." The next thing I heard was him telling the nurse that the specimen had to be sent off for a frozen section—in his words it was fifty/fifty. I felt as though somebody had just clubbed me. He told me the tumor had a hard center, which wasn't a good sign. They gave me some juice, and told me to get dressed and come back in two hours, when the biopsy report would be finished.

Those two hours were like two centuries. My husband and I sat in our car in stunned silence. I was so scared, I couldn't even cry. When we went back to Dr. Karlan's office, the minute I saw his face I knew I hadn't dodged this bullet. We sat down, and he explained the pathology report. I had lobular carcinoma. But fortunately it was in an early stage and the tumor was small.

Dr. Karlan said that tomorrow he would remove a band of tissue from around the tumor site. He was also going to remove ten lymph nodes from under my right arm, to see if the cancer had spread. The procedure, called a partial mastectomy, would be done under a general anesthetic.

I went home and sat there like a zombie. It's times like this when you really find out what you're made of. All I wanted was to survive this and get my life back as soon as possible. I felt an intense need for privacy. I called only my immediate family with the news. I just couldn't face having to relate the story over and over to each of my girlfriends. Rather, I dug deep inside myself for the strength I needed.

They say cancer is a humbling experience. I had absolutely no idea what this meant until I was diagnosed. Now I knew. When I saw homeless people on the drive back home from the city, I swear to God, I envied them. Cancer tears down your ego and destroys your confidence. I felt as though my life had been taken totally out of my own control. I might get lucky and sail through this without too much of a fight. But then again, I might not. I had no control over my own fate anymore. Maybe I never had.

"Partial mastectomy" is a scary term. But you don't lose your breast. However, they do take a good-sized chunk out. I had one big plus going for me. Since I had been an exercise fanatic for twenty years, physically I did great. The surgeries were a piece of cake for me. It was the mental torture of waiting for the next biopsy report that was nearly unbearable.

Linda and I were on the phone constantly. We were each other's lifelines for the months to come. We'd call each other every day and relate in detail what was happening with our treatments. We kept telling each other that there was a light at the end of the tunnel, and we just had to buck up and do what we had to do. But her cancer was a lot more dangerous than mine, and I knew that her scenario was not rosy. That was the tough part. Sometimes I felt as if I was giving her false hope. But then I'd think, "What the hell? Why not? She's got to be given all the hope and positive feelings possible. Her road is so much harder than mine."

I remember the first time I visited her at home, while she was going through chemotherapy. I remember how scared I was to go and see her, because I didn't want to see her weakened and suffering from the disease we both had. Although her beautiful thick black hair was mostly gone, I was really happy to see that she looked pretty darn good. She had on the gold turban I'd sent her, and was wearing makeup. We ate pizza and drank green tea, and she had a lot of her usual spunk. I was very hopeful that somehow, she was going to beat those miserable odds she had been given.

As hard as it was for me to deal with Linda's cancer, it was always harder to think about my own. Even though my case was milder, it was so much more immediate because it was happening to me. The scariest moment in my life was waiting for Dr. Karlan to give me the news from the pathologist. My lymph nodes were clear. It looked as though the cancer had spread as far as the first margin, an area around the tumor extending about one centimeter away from it. This meant I had the option of radiation treatments followed by five years of the cancer-suppressing drug tamoxifen or mastectomy with five years of tamoxifen. Tamoxifen is basically an estrogen-antagonist drug that is given to women whose tumors are estrogen-receptive, as are most breast cancers. It helps cut down the chances of recurrence of the cancer by as much as 50 percent.

Some doctors feel it's safer to have a mastectomy when the margins are not totally clear. Mine were borderline. Most of my original tumor was in situ, but it had spread in two tiny spots into the first margin that had been taken at the time of the biopsy. So, the second margin, another one centimeter taken during the partial mastectomy, showed a minimal amount of invasion—just a bit on the border. This makes it a tougher call to decide whether radiation and lumpectomy will permanently take care of it. So Dr. Karlan had me see Dr. Gary Tearston, a reconstructive surgeon, to discuss the option of a mastectomy. He also made an appointment with a woman oncologist. Between the three of us, we could decide on the right treatment for me.

Eventually I decided to undergo a double mastectomy with immediate reconstruction. A bit of overkill? Dr. Karlan thought so. He said that with radiation and six-month mammograms, he thought I'd do fine. But what was pushing me toward double mastectomy was the reality of having fibrocystic breast disease. I hated the thought of always living in fear that the other breast might develop cancer. My oncologist said that with lobular cancer, there is up to a 20 percent chance of recurrence in the other breast. I knew myself all too well. Every time a new cyst popped up, I'd be hysterical that it was the cancer returning. Also, when she examined me, the other breast was showing a cystic area. This scared the living hell out of me. I knew instinctively that I just couldn't take the anxiety of worrying about every lump, strange pain, and sore area in either breast for the rest of my life.

The second factor in choosing mastectomy was that lobular tumors are often missed on mammograms. Mine had been. They don't give off the microscopic calcium chips that the mammogram picks up from interductal cancers. Often, lobular tumors can get really big and still not show up on a mammogram. Recently, my own dermatologist developed a four-centimeter lobular tumor that was actually changing the shape of her breast, and it still wasn't showing up on a mammogram! So lobular cancer is more likely to go unnoticed by everybody. I was lucky because mine had a benign cyst on top of it and it hadn't spread into my lymph glands before we caught it. But who knew what the next time would bring?

The turning point for me was seeing a photo of a reconstructed breast in Dr. Tearston's office. He had done it on one of his nurses seven years before. She was diagnosed with breast cancer at forty-two years old, and opted for a type of reconstruction called a tram-flap. Dr. Tearston rebuilt her breast out of the fat tissue from her stomach. It looked so beautiful, I couldn't tell which breast was the reconstructed one. Actually, though, it's a much more extensive surgery than just implants, because essentially you get a tummy tuck in addition to the breast reconstruction. But because our breasts are just a bunch of fat cells anyway, a tram-flap breast has the shape, feel, look, and all the bounciness of the original.

I was floored by the naturalness of this reconstruction, but ultimately decided not to go with it. Why? Because the surgery takes about eight hours and the recovery period is several weeks, a result of the abdominal involvement. I wanted to get back to the gym and get back to normal as fast as possible. So in the end I decided against this particular surgery in favor of prosthetic implants.

Dr. Tearston told me that when one breast is rebuilt, they have to do a certain amount of work on the other breast, to get them to look symmetrical. The thought struck me immediately that if I had to have surgery on the other breast to match the reconstructed one, I'd be better off just going for implants in both. That's when I made the decision to have bilateral mastectomies with saline implants. I chose the new, more anatomically exact, teardrop-shaped implants. They just looked much closer to how my real breasts were shaped. This decision wasn't hard. Living with the fear of recurrence in the other breast, the fact that I wanted a "matched set," and the knowledge that I was doing everything I could to eliminate the cancer made the decision for bilateral mastectomies with immediate reconstruction easy.

Another bonus was that Dr. Tearston said he would be able to put the new implants in without having to use expanders. These are devices that stretch the skin around the mastectomy, so that it will be able to incorporate the implant. Sometimes a lot of skin is cut away during surgery, and it can take a few months to expand what's left. In my case, Dr. Tearston said that Dr. Karlan was a master at preserving skin, and he felt I could get away without having to have expanders. For me this was a huge psychological boost. I could wake up from the surgery exactly the same size I had been before it. The only procedure that would take a few months extra was the nipple reconstruction.

Then I had to wait five weeks for the surgery. No matter how much they reassured me, I felt that there might be cancer cells still left in my breast that might spread in those five weeks. I had the overwhelming need to just cut it all out—stat! Because I was still healing from the partial mastectomy Dr. Karlan had performed, I couldn't go to the gym, and that made me feel more helpless. But I used my treadmill, walking four miles a day until the night before surgery. The weird thing was that after the initial lumpectomy, the pain in my heel disappeared. Go figure.

Meanwhile, Linda and I talked every day. She was nearing the end of her chemo, and was hopeful that it had done its job. But her last few sessions had been incredibly rough and she was having trouble eating and swallowing. I was almost reluctant to tell her about my problems, and I finally knew what the phrase "survivor's guilt" meant. Here she was suffering physically and emotionally with no assurances that any of these efforts were going to save her life. I felt I was getting off easy, because my surgery was going to effectively give me a 90 percent chance of a cure. I felt ashamed to complain to her about my plight, because hers was a thousand times worse. Why did she have to get this type of miserable cancer? Why had she been so unlucky, and why had I caught the break? Who decides these arbitrary fates for us?

But I did talk to her, and she was incredibly supportive. Meanwhile, I tried to keep my mind occupied with my writing. Out of the blue the *Today* show called me. Matt Lauer was turning forty, and they wanted to have some fun with him. I had written a little book called *Forty—Deal with It*. The producers thought it would be fun for me to do a miniroast thing for his birthday. I was thrilled. It took my mind off everything for a while.

Today is a very professionally run show. Prior to appearing on it, I went over my material with the segment producer several times over the phone. They flew me into New York on December 29, 1997. I arrived during one hell of a storm. Normally I'd be gulping down Valium by the fistful and having mega-anxiety attacks, but *cancer changes all that*. I said to myself, "Who cares what's going on! The important thing is that I am still alive!" I was living on the most basic level. Either I was alive or I wasn't.

The show was impressive. No one knew that under my blue Tadashi suit, my chest was bandaged and there were drains in my armpit. I was determined to appear totally normal. After a few minutes of my funny little "forty" jokes, it became quite clear that Mr. Lauer was not having a good time. I guess he was having a bad-hair day or something. At one point he actually said on camera, "Who booked you on the show?" Before my cancer, I would have been rattled to the core. I would probably have caved in and let him shift the interview to a more serious vein, but not this time. Let me tell you something. I had just been through two surgeries and was facing a third *and* possibly a shortened life span. *Nobody* intimidated me—not Matt Lauer, not NBC, not all the producers in the world. I instinctively became the captain of my own ship, and nobody was going to hold a mutiny on board. I thought to myself, "This man is upset because I'm teasing him about being forty. He ought to thank God he's alive and healthy to celebrate forty." So I finished the jokes I had planned and remained undaunted. I flew back to California that afternoon.

The next day, I learned the meaning of the phrase "When it rains, it pours." My agent called to tell me that she had not been successful in her attempt to sell my manuscript. She had "lost confidence" in it. She was very sweet, but no matter how you sugarcoat it, rejection is rejection. I didn't have the heart to tell her I was awaiting cancer surgery. I've never been into giving guilt trips. So I kept quiet and politely got off the phone. But it wasn't over yet. The pièce de résistance came the following day. My son Phil called to tell me that Mr. Lauer was talking about me on the *Rosie O'Donnell Show.* And from the tone of Phil's voice, I knew Lauer wasn't giving a glowing report of me.

I tuned in to find Mr. Lauer and Rosie discussing my segment on the *Today* show. He told Rosie that he had been excited about turning forty until he found out that (1) his hairline and gum line will start receding at the same time and (2) after forty, he'll be eating so much fiber and bran, he'd have to install a seat belt on his john. My best lines!—which, remember, had been approved ahead of time by the producers.

So Rosie says, "Yeah, I saw that show. Who *was* that woman?" And Mr. Lauer says, "I don't know. Some blonde nut job. Can you believe it—she was telling fart jokes on the *Today* show!"

Now, under any other circumstances I probably would have slit my wrists on the spot. Life was not going well for me. Let's review. I just lost my agent. I was going to lose both my breasts. I was called a "nut job" by a celebrity on national TV. I was batting 0 for 3. But you know what I did? I laughed. I really didn't care. I was alive and had an excellent chance of remaining that way. And after that, all the rest of it is meaningless. Honest to God. I didn't blame Mr. Lauer. He had no idea that I was facing cancer surgery. Had he known, it might all have played out a lot differently.

Luckily, the rest of my journey was all uphill. I had the surgery on a Wednesday afternoon and went home that Friday morning. Waiting for the pathology report took over a week. That was ten times harder than the surgery. But the news was wonderful. Not one cell of residual cancer in all of the breast tissue. The tumor was small—under one centimeter. And more good news—it was not classified as a particularly aggressive cell type.

It was estrogen-receptive, so I'd be taking tamoxifen for the next five years. But because all of my test results were so good, no chemo and no radiation were necessary. I was given a 93 percent chance for survival. Can't beat those odds.

I was ecstatic. On air. I was going to live and have my chance to grow old. I thank God every day for this blessing.

I don't want to give the false impression that the surgery was a piece of cake. I was really uncomfortable for a long time. For a year, I felt as though I had two inanimate objects tightly harnessed to my chest, which is uncomfortably close to the truth. Psychologically it was really hard accepting the fact that I had been diagnosed with cancer. You want to pretend it never happened and just go back to your old life. But you can't. You are changed forever.

For the first three months after surgery, I didn't want to look at my breasts because I had no nipples. That bothered me a lot. Let's face facts. It's hard to remain in denial when you look at breasts that have no nipples. I had to wait until the mastectomy scars healed; then Dr. Tearston would create nipples from my existing skin. Even though mastectomy incisions aren't horrifying, they aren't pretty, either. Your breasts are slit from one side clear across the nipple line, down to the breastbone. Like canteloupes.

How about this? Try showering and shaving under your arms without looking at your breasts for three months! Neat trick, huh? I still don't know how the heck I did it, but I did. To avoid looking at my no-nipple breasts, I wore a T-shirt bra day and night. Obviously, I was still in a lot of denial. But that's how I coped. I still had a lot of fear. I was uncomfortable. I didn't sleep well for months. So, I'd get out my headset and listen to Art Bell all night on the radio. That's why I use so many alien-abduction jokes in my books! Then at 4 A.M. (Pacific time), I'd tune into Howard Stern and chuckle until I fell asleep at around six.

Linda and I were in touch every day. The chemo did not kill all of her tumor. She was waiting to be accepted into an experimental gene-manipulation program at UCLA. She told me that she was still hopeful that somehow she was going to be cured. But I didn't know whether she really felt that way or was just putting on a brave front. I felt even guiltier than before, because my treatments were over. I was done. I just had to heal and regain my strength. But she was fighting a battle that was getting more impossible by the day. I didn't actually get to visit her at home during this time, because she was not up to having company.

During the three weeks when she was waiting to go into the program, she was hospitalized again. She said her bowel had shut down, and even though she wasn't eating, she had put on thirty pounds. I visited her in the hospital and was shocked at her appearance. Her body was very bloated and her face looked like a chipmunk's. She didn't say so at the time, but apparently it was the swiftly growing tumors in her body that were causing the fluid retention and the weight gain.

On April 25 I wore a pretty suit and makeup to the hospital. I wanted to make sure that I looked just the way I always had. Linda and I were very close. She would know if I tried to dress down or look less healthy just to make her feel better. What made matters even sadder, it was her birthday on the twenty-eighth. I brought her some bath products, but in my heart I knew she'd never get to use them. It was just so horrific. What kind of present do you give a dying woman?

Linda went home to a hospital bed and heavy-duty medication. She was awake only a few hours a day and pretty much out of it from the painkillers. We managed to laugh a little even a week before she died. But then, during that last week, her voice got softer and softer, until one day there was no more voice. I don't know how else to describe it—she just kind of slipped away. She died in May, just eight months after her initial diagnosis.

Her death was about the worst thing I've ever experienced. Our two personas had become inextricably bound through our cancer. And now, just like that—*poof*—she was gone and I was left. Why? I felt guilty. I felt angry. But most of all, I felt really, really scared. The power of this unspeakable thing that can show up one day and arbitrarily end your life was overwhelming.

Linda and I had been friends for seven years. We shared so many of the same hopes and dreams. I never ceased to be amazed by her many and varied talents as a writer, artist, and business-woman. She was never envious of any accomplishment or good thing that came my way. It didn't diminish her. She was always so happy for my success. Even for the toughest one—that I was going to live and she probably wouldn't. But my life had to go on without her. A few weeks after the funeral, I vowed to remember Linda by having some well-deserved laughs for both of us. From the day she died, I've felt that Linda has always been with me.

When I went back to Dr. Tearston to have my nipples done, I chose to think of it as another "surgical adventure." It was a trip, all right. As Dr. Tearston was creating new nipples from the old skin, the suturing motion reminded me of my mother darning socks. Suddenly, it all seemed so funny. I watched the whole procedure in the reflection from the overhead light. I was so excited that when he finished, I said, "Houston, we've got nipples!"

Dr. Tearston thought that was a total riot. Big yuks all around the OR. When I left that day, my new nipples looked great. They should. They cost $1,500 extra! But shortly thereafter, they really swelled up. I laughed about having nipples the size of Texas. But that was okay. After a week they shrank down to the size of Rhode Island.

I must tell you, I love my new breasts. For the first time in over forty years, I can go braless and look good. They also look as though they're about six inches higher on my chest than the old ones. Hey, what do you know—I'm perky! After four years, the scars have faded nicely, so I can even flash a little cleavage if I want.

After this experience, I made sweeping changes in my life. I realized that even the specialists don't have all the answers. The doctors will monitor me for the rest of my life, but it's up to me to maintain my health. I did a lot of reading on how to stay healthy. I started eating only organically grown foods. Nothing processed—no meat, no chicken. Nothing with hormones in it. I bought a juicer. Every day, I make myself a carrot, apple, and ginger drink, which is rich in antioxidants. I eat lots of the fruits and veggies that have anticancer properties.

I meditate every day for twenty minutes, outdoors in the sunlight. I quit all the traveling. I work at maintaining as much serenity in my life as possible. I refuse to argue with anyone, anymore. No kidding. If my husband and I disagree, I go to my room and cool off for a while. Even if it takes all day for one of us to get over it, so be it. No arguing. No unkind words. I'll tell you something. When people say it's impossible to take the stress out of their lives, they're wrong. You can. I'm living proof that you can.

I also drink a lot more water than I used to. I still exercise six days a week. I work at staying healthy and happy. The one thing I came away from my experience knowing was this: It's the denial that kills women more often than the cancer. A Stage I breast cancer is a whole different animal from a Stage III. Early detection makes a huge difference in dealing with cancer.

That's why I *can't stress enough* how important it is to have a mammogram every year. Even then, mammograms miss 15 percent of all breast cancers, so that's why examining your breasts every month is so important. The key is to look for asymmetry. Because I was so familiar with the geography of my breasts, I was able to tell when there was a change.

Please don't wait for a whole year to have your doctor do a breast exam for you. It might make the difference between living and dying. Look at your breasts in front of a mirror. Check the skin for any possible changes in color, texture, or shape. If you feel anything, do not take a wait-and-see posture. When you become aggressive about taking charge of your own breasts, it will give you a wonderful feeling of empowerment in your life.

There have been some phenomenal advances in the treatment of breast cancer in the last five years. The chemotherapies and treatments like stem-cell transplants are incredibly effective. Nowadays, women are not dying two years after diagnosis as they once did—even when they're in the more advanced stages. My wonderful friend Carlynn Donosky was diagnosed five years ago with a Stage II. She had three positive lymph nodes, so her chances of survival were a lot lower than if she had just two positive. She never cried. She did her homework, learning as much as she could about Stage II interductal breast cancer. She had double mastectomies with immediate reconstruction and four months of chemo, and took the five-year regimen of tamoxifen. She never missed a day during chemo being sick. She said she was slightly "queasy" and had a metallic taste in her mouth. But that was it! No vomiting. No days spent in bed. She made smart choices. She even had a hysterectomy a few years after her mastectomies for added insurance, because her tumor was estrogen-receptive. This would further lower any estrogen in her system. The fact that she was past menopause made that decision easier to make. And because she so unselfishly shared every step of her experience with me, I had a better knowledge of what to do when it was my turn. Last month, Carlynn joyfully celebrated five years of cancer-free life. Way to go, babe. Love you.

Most cancer patients live with a certain amount of fear that the cancer may return someday. I'll admit, it's not an idyllic way to go through the rest of your life. But I'll tell you something.

Nobody appreciates their life more than a cancer survivor. We could give seminars about living in the minute! I try to live in that 93 percent zone, continually reminding myself that my odds are excellent for remaining cancer-free. And every year, medical science is that much closer to coming up with a cure. It gives so much hope for everyone.

Because I have learned how to love and care for my body, I am enjoying excellent health. I have a wonderful new publisher, a trusted friend as my new literary agent, a flourishing career, a happy marriage, and the world's greatest sons. My grandchildren light up my life brighter than any star in the sky. I give thanks to God every day for having been able to recover so quickly and get my life back.

Hey, not bad for a "blonde nut job," huh?